How to Succeed on Primary Care and Community Placements

This title is also available as an e-book.
For more details, please see
www.wiley.com/buy/9781118343449
or scan this QR code:

How to Succeed on Primary Care and Community Placements

David Pearson

General Practitioner, Yorkshire
Director, Academy of Primary Care
Hull York Medical School
Universities of Hull and York
York, UK

Sandra Nicholson

Lead, Academic Unit for Community-Based Medical Education
Barts and The London School of Medicine and Dentistry
Queen Mary University of London
London, UK

WILEY Blackwell

Library of Congress Cataloging-in-Publication Data

Pearson, David (David J.), author.
  How to succeed on primary care and community placements / David Pearson, Sandra Nicholson.
    p. ; cm.
  Includes bibliographical references and index.
  ISBN 978-1-118-34344-9 (pbk.)
I. Nicholson, Sandra, author.   II. Title.
[DNLM: 1. Primary Health Care–Great Britain.   2. Clinical Clerkship–Great Britain.
3. Community Health Services–Great Britain.   4. Education, Medical,
Undergraduate–Great Britain. W 84.6]
  RA427
  362.120941–dc23
                                              2015026509
A catalogue record for this book is available from the British Library.

Wiley also publishes its books in a variety of electronic formats. Some content that appears in print may not be available in electronic books.

Cover image: Meaden Creative

Set in 10/13pt Minion by SPi Global, Pondicherry, India

Printed in Singapore by C.O.S. Printers Pte Ltd

1 2016

Contents

Chapter 6: Learning medicine in community settings, 111

With Ann O'Brien and Will Spiring

Chapter 7: Clinical information systems, opportunities to learn, 128

With Jane Kirby

Chapter 8: Supporting learning in primary care using social media and other technologies, 151

With Jonathon Tomlinson

Chapter 9: Assessment, feedback and quality assurance, 167

With Mark Williamson

Contributors

Maria Hayfron-Benjamin
Lecturer in Medical Education
Barts and The London School of
Medicine and Dentistry
Queen Mary University of
London
London

Jane Kirby
Academic Unit of Primary Care
University of Leeds School of
Medicine

Catie Nagel
GP & Course Director iBSc
Primary Care
Academic Unit of Primary Care
Leeds Institute of Health Sciences
University of Leeds

Ann O'Brien
Clinical Senior Lecturer
Barts and The London School of
Medicine and Dentistry
Queen Mary University of
London
London

Will Spiring
Clinical Teaching Fellow,
Community Based Medical
Education
Barts and The London School of
Medicine and Dentistry
Queen Mary University of London
London

Jonathon Tomlinson
NIHR in Practice Research
Fellow
Queen Mary University of London
London

Mark Williamson
Academic Lead for Primary Care
Education
Hull York Medical School
York

Introduction

International healthcare systems, including a modernised NHS within the United Kingdom, increasingly need clinicians in the future who have the appropriate knowledge and skills to work in community settings. Community-based clinical care is changing rapidly, with the increasing movement of patient care from hospital to community settings, there is an increased reliance on clinical information systems, clinical guidelines and protocols and more emphasis on highly organised team-based care for patients with long-term conditions. For example, in the United Kingdom the Department of Health expects 50% of the future NHS workforce to practise in the community (DoH, 2013). Future doctors, such as you, need to have education tailored to address the changing needs of the future clinical environment and how clinical care will be provided for patients. Medical education is seeking new ways of workplace-based learning, revisiting apprenticeship models and exploring new assessment models. Our book acknowledges and addresses these new realities and is equally relevant to you and your tutors.

This book provides the information you as medical students need to know to get the most out of your community-based placements. Most UK-based medical students will begin to attend community placements from their first year of studies and it is important that you know what to expect and how to maximise your learning opportunities. You may otherwise miss out on essential clinical learning that balances and brings alive both your medical school theoretical teaching and learning from placements in other clinical settings.

'Community-based placements' is a loose generalised term to describe any of your clinical placements that occur outside of a university or hospital setting. The first port of call for most patients worldwide seeking help with their health concerns will be services based in the community. Frequently, medical school placements will be organised within primary care settings using members of the primary healthcare team as your tutors. Within a UK context primary care services focussing on general practice and the immediate practice-based team are common placements. The detail will vary across other healthcare systems. Wider community placements with voluntary organisations, specialist tertiary centres and outreach clinics may also be available.

This book has been written by experienced general practitioners and educators, closely involved with delivering community-based education, and aims to be a practical guide for undergraduate medical community placements. It has primarily been written for you as students, although you may find it helpful to share some of it with your tutors and we hope they will also find much in here of direct interest. It isn't written only for students wishing to be GPs. On the contrary, we strongly believe all future doctors can learn much of their medical knowledge in community settings and for those set on a career in hospital medicine or surgery, this book and community experiences provide a vital insight into the care provided to your future patients across most of their lives. The book aims to inspire you about community medicine, provides an insight into learning about clinical medicine including teamwork and also medical specialty teaching relevant to a community setting. As such, unique elements of community-based teaching ranging from clinical information systems to home visits are included.

Each chapter is written with considerable student and tutor input; ensuring chapters are fresh, relevant and up to date. Where possible you are encouraged to read and learn actively and each chapter describes its learning outcomes at the start with reference to tasks for you to reinforce what you may learn on placement. Community-based medical education isn't just about a change in location. Many students find that they have opportunities to engage in very personal learning with individual tutor attention and focussed feedback across a range of clinical and non-clinical community settings. We have tried to ensure this is a practical guide that will allow you to best work with your tutors to make your time in community settings informative and inspiring.

Many medical schools now use community-based medical education to cover a significant component of their undergraduate curriculum, reflecting the changing nature of healthcare worldwide, the increasing importance of recognising the social determinants of health, and the challenge of meeting the costs associated with healthcare. Rapidly changing patient demographics, an ageing global population, advances in medical treatment and a consequent expansion in multi-morbidity and complexity of care worldwide have highlighted the importance of community care.

What can you expect as you read the book?

Chapter 1 explains what you can learn within your community placements in early years, including the psycho-social determinants of health, and how clinical placements within primary care emphasise the holistic longitudinal nature of patients' conditions, which highlight a multi-professional team-based approach. We explore clinical placements from early years teaching that introduces patients and related clinical material alongside your theoretical medical science teaching, middle year placements that focus on learning clinical method, communication and clinical skills, to later placements specifically designed to learn aspects of clinical and specialty medicine common to the community, such as the management of long-term medical conditions. These later placements also give opportunities to prepare for the transition to more independent practice, so we focus on aspects of professionalism and continuing professional development. Chapter 2 gives an introduction to the opportunities available to learn about public health aspects of medicine, and the chance to learn about health prevention and promotion at individual, community and regional levels. Chapter 3 explores how best to learn within community settings. It includes some very practical advice that you need to consider before embarking upon these placements, including what necessary preparations you should make that will both ensure that you are safe and that you get the most out of your time. Chapter 4 explores the centrality of the doctor–patient interaction and what you can learn from the process of a GP consultation.

Chapter 5 widens your learning opportunities. It introduces the primary healthcare team, what you can learn from individual members, how such a team works to deliver and improve patient care. We explore how medicines are prescribed and managed within community settings (something that offers many opportunities for you to learn about not only pharmacology but also the underlying medical conditions and the issues that many patients raise regarding co-morbidity and multiple drug use). The chapter includes what we can learn from patients themselves and how you can best involve patients directly in your learning. Chapter 6 looks at how our patient care is delivered within wider community settings and teams, including the learning opportunities from visits to patients' homes and residential care homes and also learning from the professionals, who make up the wider community-based health teams. It explores various aspects of preventive and public health, including women and children's services, mental health and palliative and end of life care. The chapter also includes examples and ideas for learning outside of health settings with voluntary and community support groups.

Chapters 7 and 8 are a little more specialised. Detailed clinical information systems, information technology, patient records are included in Chapter 7, and it also describes advice on planning your audit, quality improvement and research projects. Chapter 8 describes in some detail what opportunities and challenges new advances in technology and social media provide to enhance learning; especially with regards to e-learning and social media. Chapter 9 explains how you may be assessed during the placement and the importance of two-way feedback, that is, from your tutors to you and from you back to your placements. We also offer tips on how to get the most out of your placement and learn from these assessments.

Finally, Chapter 10 reflects on the journey we have taken and you are just beginning to describe some of the future and currently developing aspects of community-based learning.

We hope you enjoy and find this book helpful in preparing for and getting the most out of your community placements. Most of all we hope that you learn what it is that you need to know in becoming an excellent, engaged and empathic doctor and make the most out of the opportunities for learning from your community placements.

Reference

Department of Health (2013) Delivering high quality, effective, compassionate care: Developing the right people with the right skills and the right values. A mandate from the Government to Health Education England: April 2013 to March 2015. http://hee.nhs.uk/wp-content/uploads/sites/321/2013/11/HEE-Mandate.pdf. Accessed July 11, 2015.

Acknowledgements

We would like to offer sincere thanks to the following:

Those contributors who wrote chapters for us or with us. Without you the book would have been much narrower, one-dimensional and diminished. Striking a balance between *carte blanche* and conformity is never easy – we hope we managed it and that you are as satisfied with the final outcome as we are.

Our various student writers and reviewers who, especially at the outset, gave us direction and guidance about what was important to you – you encouraged us to be more practical and less academic in our approach.

We thank all our student contributors who contributed their insight, ideas and comments to this work, especially Jenny Macallan and Jeeves Wijesuriya (both now qualified as doctors).

Various reviewers and critical friends. We couldn't take on board all the comments, but all were discussed – and we did try!

Our publishers for their great patience through various crises and periods of contemplation.

Finally, colleagues in our respective medical schools who at various times gave us space, encouragement, advice or a gentle prod to get it done. We finally did so – thank you.

David Pearson
Sandra Nicholson

Chapter 1 **What to learn in community settings**

With Ann O'Brien

Introduction

Medicine is best learned from patients, and patients overwhelmingly engage with healthcare in their own community settings. Increasingly modern healthcare is structured to occur in community settings, and it necessarily follows that much of medicine can, and we believe should, be learned in these settings. This chapter highlights aspects of the undergraduate syllabus common to many medical schools that you will have the chance to learn in primary care and the community as you progress through your undergraduate curriculum. In Chapter 2 we focus particularly on public health and health promotion aspects of medicine, and in later chapters we explore the practicalities.

Helping you appreciate all that you can learn while on a community placement will motivate you to make the most of your time. This is important because some topics will only be covered during your time in the community and hence it's useful for you to know how these learning opportunities may present. There are additionally many opportunities for you to see how community-based medical education complements and puts into perspective the science and theoretical learning you do at university and also your hospital-based experiences.

How to Succeed on Primary Care and Community Placements, First Edition.
David Pearson and Sandra Nicholson.
© 2016 John Wiley & Sons, Ltd. Published 2016 by John Wiley & Sons, Ltd.

2 **Primary care and community placements**

By the end of this chapter you should be able to:
- be aware of what areas of your curriculum can be covered within the community
- understand how early attachments lay the foundations for later clinical placements
- appreciate how this book will help support you to make the most of such learning opportunities

Making the most of your community time whether you eventually become a general practitioner (GP), hospital physician or surgeon is time well spent as what you learn in this setting will make you better clinicians.

It is important that medical students receive clinical experience in a range of healthcare settings. The healthcare system in the UK is varied, increasingly decentralised and subject to change. A varied medical education and clinical experience can help students adapt to these differences and changes when they graduate. Clinical placements should start early in the undergraduate curriculum.

Furthermore:

Placements should reflect the changing patterns of healthcare and must provide experience in a variety of environments including hospitals, general practices and community medical services.

(GMC Tomorrow's Doctors, 2009)

This chapter is divided into four sections: early years, middle years, later years and further opportunities which reflect the range of community attachments occurring within an undergraduate medical curriculum. Each section outlines what you and your tutors might expect such a placement, at that time of the curriculum, to deliver. You will have different opportunities depending on how your medical school delivers its curriculum, but there is often a common core syllabus with similar aims and learning objectives. Although much of this book focuses on a UK perspective, the principles and many examples are of relevance if you are a student studying outside of the United Kingdom. Community placements are designed to provide increasing clinical exposure and responsibility across the years as you become more knowledgeable. Equally the concept of longitudinal integrated clerkships (LICs) is gathering momentum in medical education; primary and community care will tend to have a disproportionate role in delivering these longitudinal experiences and the advantages they are thought to bring. Ultimately all these placements aim to help you to prepare for independent clinical practice.

Take a look at what some of the world's leading medical educationalists have to say about what competencies a doctor should have (CanMEDS Framework; http://www.royalcollege.ca/portal/page/portal/rc/canmeds/framework) or what the UK's General Medical Council has to say (http://www.gmc-uk.org/education/undergraduate/tomorrows_doctors.asp):

> The curriculum will include practical experience of working with patients throughout all years, increasing in duration and responsibility so that graduates are prepared for their responsibilities as provisionally registered doctors. It will provide enough structured clinical placements to enable students to demonstrate the 'outcomes for graduates' across a range of clinical specialties, including at least one student assistantship period.
>
> GMC (2009) Tomorrow's Doctors; Para 84

Early years

Meeting patients, learning how and why some people become ill, and how to help them were some of the reasons why you wanted to become doctors. The social and psychological aspects of health and illness are well covered during community attachments. You will therefore be able to learn about how patients' lives and work affect their health and experience of disease.

This is one of the important learning outcomes stated by GMC:

> Explain sociological factors that contribute to illness, the course of the disease and the success of treatment including issues relating to health inequalities, the links between occupation and health and the effects of poverty and affluence.
>
> GMC (2009) Tomorrow's Doctors:
> Outcomes 1 The doctor as scholar and a scientist

TASK

Why not take another look at the GMC's document 'Tomorrow's Doctors, 2009' or its equivalent alternatives such as the Scottish Doctor or the CanMEDS (for links, see reference section) and see what you need to know and what can be covered during your community placements.

Meeting your first patient as a medical student can seem daunting, and you may also feel that your patient may have unrealistic expectations of what you know and can do. Early patient contact often occurs within primary care and the community and sets a student's mind at ease, increases your confidence and begins to make you feel like you are learning to be a real doctor, ensuring your theoretical knowledge is grounded in a patient-centred holistic framework.

> Early on, it is easy to fixate on skills you think you lack, or believe that you must have answers for the patient, or be able to diagnose illness. In reality, this is an opportunity to develop innate skills that underpin this diagnostic ability. Learning how to talk to patients, empathise with their problems and appreciate the impact of illness on their life without a diagnostic or history taking agenda may be the most valuable thing you develop in your entire medical career.
>
> (Final year medical student)

What to learn during early patient contact

Community placements are an opportunity for you to meet patients early on. Often referred to as early patient contact (EPC), these placements focus on authentic patient interactions, encourage you to appreciate the psycho-social aspects of medicine and contribute to your growing understanding of the varying roles of different health professionals involved in multi-professional team working (Dornan and Bundy, 2004). Opportunities will be available for you to actively engage with patients in a safe clinical environment, helping you to reflect on developing your communication skills and attitudes towards patients and illness. This is an important task which should complement your growing scientific knowledge. Becoming a doctor requires you to learn from a structured curriculum that balances learning to know with learning to care.

Benefits of early patient contact:
- Brings alive your scientific learning
- Encourages confidence in students
- Sets the scene for later clinical learning
- Develops a patient-centred approach

TASK

Introduce yourself to a patient by explaining who you are and that you would like to find out how their health affects them. Consider how you should best approach this interaction with a patient and whether there are any ethical issues involved such as confidentiality.

Community-based EPC provides you with a learning environment which integrates scientific and clinical education. With a more holistic view of medicine you will be able to better appreciate the clinical context of the underlying biomedical principles you are learning about elsewhere (Dahle *et al.*, 2002). Your early clinical exposure contextualises the science you need to learn in order to fully understand the clinical scenarios, which you will engage with later on in your training (Dornan and Bundy, 2004). If you have been enthusiastic and engaged with earlier clinical opportunities that highlight the centrality of patients, you will feel better prepared and more confident when you start your clinical placements later. Primary care often reflects opportunities to meet with patients, who in their own environments, feel empowered to talk with you, and share their experiences with you, more so than when they are hospitalised.

TASK

Speak to your community tutor. Explain what you have recently covered at medical school. Your tutors should understand the content of your curriculum but their experiences at medical school may be very different compared to yours. Then discuss how the medical science that you are learning can be applied to the clinical situations you see each day.

Professionalism and personal growth

Learning to be a doctor requires more than just factual knowledge or even the application of the appropriate clinical skills. It requires the embodiment of attitudes and behaviours akin to being a professional doctor. Being a good doctor is about who you are, how you treat your patients and colleagues, and how you recognise your own shortcomings and do something about them. Your early community placements will give you time to observe good professional behaviour in a variety of healthcare professionals. Your tutors will also help you think through why you wouldn't want to copy some behaviour, which you think is not good.

TASK

Take a moment to think about what it means to be a doctor. Look up what the General Medical Council (GMC) has published about what is expected concerning the professional standards of doctors. Their publication 'Good Medical Practice (GMP)' will help you think more deeply. This can be accessed from http://www.gmc-uk.org/guidance/good_medical_practice.asp

---

It's never too early to have read through the statements made in the UK GMC's guidance on what it means to be a good doctor outlined in GMP. You will be able to see ethical dilemmas (http://www.gmc-uk.org/gmpinaction/) and be able to discuss with both your tutors and peers the issues involved. Similarly if and when issues of conflict arise you will have the chance to learn from these situations and think about the theoretical principles you have learned in the classroom.

Each section of this chapter outlines areas of the syllabus covered within the community that can specifically help you learn how to become a good doctor. Early contact, with patients and healthcare teams, sets the scene for you in your early training and provides essential medical role models. Think about who it is you wish to emulate and also which behaviour or attitude that you would not wish to copy and why?

This environment whether good or bad offers a variety of examples from which you can derive good practice. Every good or bad example one encounters (though in an ideal world they are all good) should be analysed and reflected on to help you adapt your practice to the ideal you hope to attain. When you see a patient confused as management has not been clearly explained, this is an example of how important it is to take the time to go through things that might not necessarily seem complex to you, but can to a patient. Even negative experiences can be used for positive change to your practice

(Final year student)

Early patient contact provides exposure to real ethical and medico-social dilemmas which you can explore with your tutors. These opportunities raise the potential to integrate your theoretical teaching with real world medicine. A wide variety of domains of medical professionalism are appropriate for you to have practical experience of and learn about during your early community placements. Direct EPC brings these into stark relief compared to classroom teaching. For example, the demonstration of respect for patients (or an ability to reflect on its absence), modelling of good teamwork and leadership, the reinforcement of seeing how doctors' social responsibilities are actually put into practice, are all useful and very practical day-to-day issues that you will come across in the community (see also Hilton, 2004). Being honest with patients and admitting what you don't know, but how you will deal with this and still help them, is one of the earliest aspects of medical professionalism you will need to learn.

Medical professionalism:
- Central to being a good doctor
- Early patient contact provides opportunities to experience professional challenges
- Reflect on good role models

Early community placements also provide ample opportunity for encouraging and practising reflection, essential skills for lifelong learning in medicine. Reflection – the conscious weighing and integrating of views from different perspectives – is a necessary prerequisite for becoming a safe and successful medical professional. Reflecting on educational and clinical experiences in medical practice, including one's own behaviour, is crucial (Boenink *et al.*, 2004). Early patient contact gives you authentic material to reflect on early in your careers. Tutors can encourage and support this process.

TASK

Ask your tutors to help you reflect by sharing and discussing any reflective learning logs that you are commonly asked to complete during your attachments. Consider discussing with your peers or other learners, together in small groups, your draft reflective writing.

Community-based teaching often occurs in small groups and allows individual feedback. Discussing cases and your experiences with other students helps you reflect and also gather a consensus opinion about what is the 'right thing to do'. However remember to maintain patients' confidentiality – no names or other patient-identifiable data, and consider the environment for such a discussion, probably not the bus on the way home.

Patient perspectives on health and healthcare

Seeing patients from the very beginning of your training provides early opportunities to explore what patients believe about health and illness. You should consider how patients' beliefs may affect what and when patients present with their symptoms, and which symptoms warrant a patient even wishing to see a doctor. GPs are true general physicians and these attachments are an ideal opportunity to understand how patients' views affect both their diagnosis and treatment. You will be able to see first-hand how GPs and other healthcare professionals influence patient compliance with medication, long-term follow-up and adherence to management plans.

> Patients come from different backgrounds and all sorts of walks of life. It is remarkable the health beliefs and lifestyle practices patients can have! Talking to patients from different walks of life can give you an appreciation of the different things people can believe and an insight into different walks of life
>
> (Final year medical student)

Seeing patients within their own homes and communities gives you a particularly unique and valuable opportunity to understand the complexity of health and illness and what effect they have on patients' lives. The relevance of cultural and social perspectives that influence patients' health beliefs, are highlighted within this context (Helman, 2007). Learning medical science within a community clinical context will help you develop a social awareness. Understanding why patients present with symptoms when they do, and what expectations they have of the healthcare service they receive, will help you develop a patient-centred model of practicing medicine. Understanding how patients' expectations of different healthcare professionals vary and how this affects who they visit, and what services they use, should encourage you to visit, and learn about, a variety of community services available in your area.

Some medical undergraduate curricula use LICs to foster within medical students a greater sense of the patient being at the centre of the care that they receive. LICs depend on medical students having the opportunities to follow individual patients as they access a variety of healthcare services and interact with the patient through the stages of presentation, investigation, diagnosis, referral and treatment. Community services present appropriate settings for LICs acting as the focal point even as patients access hospital and tertiary care, as required (Ogur and Hirsh, 2009).

TASK

You will have plenty of opportunities to observe healthcare professionals talking with patients. Use this time to consider which aspects of their consultation styles foster a patient-centred approach and how this can benefit both patients and the healthcare professional. Listen to how patients' ideas, concerns and expectations are elicited and addressed.

Social and psychological aspects of health

Medical graduates should be able to: Explain sociological factors that contribute to illness, the course of the disease and the success of treatment – including issues relating to health inequalities, the links between occupation and health and the effects of poverty and affluence.

Tomorrow's doctors (2009) Para 10 (d)

The UK GMC recommends that medical students appreciate both the social and psychological impact of illness on patients' lives and the close association between sociological factors and the onset of ill health. In community placements you will see first-hand how a variety of issues may have an impact on health, for example, poverty, unemployment and homelessness. Attachments to voluntary organisations while on community placements, or GPs with interests in specific areas, such as homeless patients can widen your experience and understanding of how socioeconomic deprivation may affect health. For example, you will notice that many patients seen in community placements, such as homeless shelters may also have drug, alcohol or mental health problems. Why is that? Debate the connection with your community tutor or fellow students. Identify the factors in the patient's 'life history', for example level of education, employment history, social class, family background, cultural background, which impacts their illness experience and coping mechanisms.

Key psycho-social aspects:
• Understanding how the health beliefs of patients may affect their attitude and behaviour towards illness and healthcare
• Appreciating the significant socio-demographic determinants of health and illness

---

Take a look at the United Nation's 8 World Development Goals (http://www.un.org/millenniumgoals/). In September 2000 world leaders came together at United Nations Headquarters in New York to form a new global partnership which aims to reduce extreme poverty with a series of time-bound targets that have become known as the Millennium Development Goals. These initiatives highlight how healthcare is defined by more than just discrete illness, it is multi-factorial. In the United Kingdom and worldwide, the individual's living condition, education, opportunities and support system are huge factors that affect a person's health. Try to explore a real timeline of patients, from birth to date, to really understand the impact of the social setting upon patients' health.

Early clinical placements will allow you to explore from the start of your career how similar medical conditions can affect different patients

---

TASK

Early placements in general practice and the community provide numerous opportunities for you to begin practice by taking social histories from patients. Take the opportunity. Consider how the information you have gleaned may have affected the patient's health. Consider how they cope with their illness and treatment options. Discuss and consider why this information is important with your tutors.

in different ways at different times. Also you will learn about why people might become ill and how housing, poverty, loneliness, poor diet, employment and crime might affect health and vice versa.

> Take the time to explore a patient's living situation and take note of the adaptations they have made to their daily life to cope with their illness. Often these changes go unmentioned as they have become second nature but you can often spot real challenges they face! Moreover you can see the impact simple home additions from occupational therapy can have!
>
> (Final year student)

TIP

Try and see and talk with as many patients from diverse backgrounds as possible. Explain to patients and seek their consent to discuss with them their social, cultural or psychological background. Talk to colleagues in confidence. Why is it important we know this background?

Learning clinical method (history taking and examination)

At the beginning of your clinical training you will take a long time to take a full history and fully examine a patient. There will be opportunities for you to do this individually and often in pairs within community settings. The components and the communication processes underpinning taking a professional and coherent full history can be learned and practised within general practice. You will have an opportunity to receive feedback from your tutors and peers, which you can use to improve your clinical skills. General practice also has a long history of using recorded consultations in learning and teaching; seize this opportunity if you are offered it – you will find watching yourself conduct histories – an invaluable learning tool.

Students, who have specific sessions within general practice, may have several patients invited for an afternoon to be clerked by you; students take turns to interview and examine patients in an agreed sequence. These sessions are often themed to cover specific learning objectives from modules.

TIP: GETTING THE MOST OUT OF SEEING PATIENTS

If you are currently undertaking a cardiorespiratory module and patients have been invited for you to interview and examine, it would be expected that you understood which broad question areas to explore with patients, for example, asking about chest pain, breathlessness and cough. In addition you should have read through an examination guide that introduces how to examine the cardiac and respiratory systems.

You will not be expected to do these tasks at a consultant level from the start but anticipating the basics means that you can make the most of your time with the patients and learn from the GP tutor. So, clinical methods can be learned in general practice from the very beginning of your medical training with simple histories and very basic examinations to start with, building up to full patient clerking during your clinical years and then honing your skills before finals in the later years. Overall, the main emphasis will be on learning about medicine within the context of your patients' lives.

Now is the time not only to consolidate taking a routine history and performing an appropriate examination but also to consider how the patient's symptoms and signs fit within the context of a more holistic appreciation of medicine. This means developing your understanding of what fosters a patient-centred approach, and how your knowledge and skills in gathering relevant information and eliciting signs from patients, needs to then lead onto formulating a shared management plan with patients.

Flick through common examinations before firms so when you have to do one you have an idea of what to do fresh in your mind!

(Final year medical student)

General practice is a great place for seeing patients with multiple and diverse medical conditions. Many medical schools have introduced portfolios for you to complete as you progress through each academic year. Portfolios help you to prepare for the types of assessments and self-evaluations you will need to complete as doctors. More information about portfolios and the kind of documentation and reflection that you can include from your time in general practice is discussed in Chapter 9.

Clinical and procedural skills

> Be Proactive! Lots of surgeries take bloods for testing and have
> specific phlebotomy clinics. Offer yourself up to take bloods! A day
> spent doing this is never wasted! The same with Flu jabs in the
> winter!
>
> (Final year medical student)

Many near-patient tests and other investigations occur within the
general practice setting and many of these will be required to be signed
off for your portfolios. Being hands-on with practical medical skills
increases your confidence and helps make you feel part of the team.
Most of the following can be achieved in general practice sessions:
Urinalysis
Blood pressure reading
Peak flow and spirometry
Electrocardiogram (ECG, performing and reading)
Subcutaneous and intramuscular injections
Venepuncture
Minor operations such as cryotherapy

Often GP surgeries run clinics where patients come in purely for
these tests, injections or to have their blood taken, and it is a great place
to learn and practice these skills. Often, given the size of the list, they
welcome your help completing these lists yourself once trained in that
skill. We will explore this in more detail in Chapter 5.

TASK

Sit with your tutor and consider the practical and procedural skills you need
to learn.

Are there any gaps? If so plan how to get these done while in general practice.

Having a completed portfolio will be a really satisfying way to finish your
attachment!

NB *Whilst you will start learning clinical history taking, examination
and skills in early years you will continually revisit them and hone
these skills across the years at medical school. The learning doesn't stop at
graduation either!*

Middle clinical years

Learning clinical medicine in primary care

In the middle years of your training you will spend the majority of your time within a clinical setting. Often this will be in an acute medical environment, such as hospital wards and outpatient clinics. However, time within the community, such as GP placements and other outreach clinics, complements your experience and is an important component of your education. It is important that you make the most of this time. The way care is delivered to patients has radically changed over the past 10 years with more and more patients being diagnosed and treated solely within the community. This indicates not only a significant increase in the diversity of workload for primary care physicians within developed countries but also a greater provision of community health services worldwide. With an ageing population, advanced healthcare worldwide, and the increasingly recognised importance of health promotion and the prevention of diseases, your community-based education is therefore a very important component of your clinical experience. Some have argued that 'the future of a sustainable health system would seem to rest in primary care as never before' (Barker, 2010).

Most patients' care is predominately coordinated within the community. Hospitals, secondary care services and specialised tertiary referral centres are good learning opportunities to see the acutely unwell patients and those who require specialist care, but your learning also needs to be focused on where the majority of patients are found, and how their conditions are managed. General practice and community settings provide invaluable opportunities to see patients with long-term medical conditions who are well enough to spend time with you discussing their presentation, symptoms and management, and most importantly are likely to be prepared to be examined. Furthermore you will miss out and not see a variety of clinical conditions nor appreciate how patients are appropriately managed if your only exposure to patients is within acute settings. Community attachments provide essential opportunities for you to learn and participate in patient care that is designed to occur within the context of patients' lives. This emphasises the importance of home, work, carers and overall the practice of medicine that has at its heart patient-centredness. For example, middle-year clinical experiences often provide attachments for medical students to learn about contraception, community antenatal clinics to better understand the routine care provided for pregnant women, and attachments to hospices, or voluntary nursing services, that care for the terminally ill within their own homes and communities.

The management of common long-term conditions such as cardio-vascular diseases, obstructive airways diseases, asthma and diabetes are good examples of where patients may never be seen within a hospital setting but have a significant morbidity that is managed successfully within the community. This is a worldwide phenomenon as long-term conditions become more prevalent and 'health care systems worldwide are faced with the challenge of responding to the needs of people with chronic medical conditions such as diabetes, heart failure and mental illness' (World Health Organization, 2002).

Your placement in primary care and community settings will, therefore, help you understand how care within the community is organised and relates to the secondary care hospital services. There will be opportunities to engage with patients who present with acute symptoms, understand the variety of initial presentations of new long-term diagnoses, and how primary care gives you a unique insight into how to differentiate between common non-serious conditions and possible significant pathology.

General practice attachments provide opportunities to see patients with common conditions, both acute and long-term, that have not presented during your highly specialised hospital firms. Primary care in particular presents many opportunities for you to learn from patients not only about their conditions but also about how these conditions are individually best managed.

Long-term conditions are diagnosed and are actively managed in the community – only referring to secondary services for specialist investigation or advice. These represent a significant proportion of the workload of community healthcare professionals. Some of the most important common long-term conditions that you will see in general practice are as follows:

Osteoarthritis, backache and other joint problems
Hypertension
Coronary artery disease, angina and heart failure

Asthma and chronic obstructive pulmonary disease
Diabetes and its complications
Chronic renal failure
Thyroid disease
Inflammatory bowel conditions
Skin conditions, such as eczema, psoriasis
Mental health conditions, such as depression, dementia
If your medical school hasn't emphasised which conditions you should prioritise then talk to your GP tutor to plan how best to utilise your time. Most student concerns originate from either not being given the opportunity to clerk patients themselves or that the 'right' patients are unavailable. As the majority of illness and its management occurs in the community you should have ample opportunities to see patients. Take a proactive approach and make the most of the opportunities that arise for you to see, talk with and examine patients that present. This includes at this stage exploring how their condition is managed and how this affects them, their families and work. If you do feel that you aren't seeing the appropriate patients then you do need to discuss this with your GP tutor and also your central department if issues are not resolved.

> There are lots of illnesses to learn about and they can seem daunting and complex. By reinforcing how to learn about illness with an understanding and relationship with a real patient, you can develop an in depth long-term understanding of not only the illness and its symptoms and management, but also the complications of treatment, risk factors and its potential impact of the other aspects of daily life
> (Final-year student)

While medical schools will have articulated a community timetable that fits with your university and hospital teaching modules, do not let this dissuade you from seeing patients who present acutely with new, interesting symptoms and possibly accompanying signs. In many countries, primary care physicians act as the gateway to other care, encouraging a coordinated patient-centred approach. Many patients who develop a serious illness initially present to a family doctor. You will therefore have many opportunities to see and understand how GPs evaluate patients' symptoms and differentiate between minor self-limiting illness and possible significant morbidity, and begin to do this for yourselves. Sick patients come to the GP and you need to appreciate how best to recognise these patients and how to help them. Many attachments will have opportunities for you to attend 'out of hours' and emergency work. This will also stand you in good stead when you are later asked to assess acutely unwell patients on the wards.

Examples of common acute conditions are febrile illness such as upper respiratory infections, chest infections, possibly urinary tract infections and simple ENT conditions. Knowing how to recognise these conditions and being able to offer simple advice is essential and will make you feel like a proper doctor. Acute abdominal pain is a common condition, and knowing how to quickly assess such a patient and be able to differentiate between the possible multiple common non-serious causes while also excluding the more significant conditions is necessary.

TASK

Look up and reflect upon 'red flag symptom and signs' that GPs look out for. These indicate the possible presence of serious pathology, sometimes cancer, and encourage primary care physicians to consider referring these patients on to specialist services and/or further investigation.

See, for example, http://www.gponline.com/education/medical-red-flags.

What guidance is there to help healthcare practitioners decide what to do? Understanding the underlying principles that dictate the speed and route of entry to secondary care isn't about making you into GPs, but helping you recognise significant symptoms, disease progression and appropriate standards of management. Observing initially when you first come to general practice is an amazing chance to see a whole consultation; introduction, presentation of the history, examination and management plan including possible investigations and treatment. An opportunity to see everything all together! Chapter 4 goes into more depth concerning what you can learn about and during the consultation. However for now let's have a further look at how you can practise specific clinical skills within general practice.

Learning about specialities in primary care

Students commonly have rotations through different medical and surgical specialties during their penultimate clinical year. General practice attachments during these rotations give you insight into the common presentations and long-term management of conditions found within these specialties, and inform you of how generalists and specialists work together to care for patients. There are several areas that you really will only see nowadays in the community, for example, the routine normal care of pregnant women and the surveillance of normal child development. Although your hospital firms will give you excellent exposure to the potential acute illness that infrequently occurs during pregnancy and childhood and teach you how to investigate, diagnose and treat these conditions, it is essential that you appreciate what is normal and physiological first. Thereafter you can begin to learn about what can go wrong and how best to diagnose and manage common conditions that relate to the medical specialties that usually first present in the community.

Child health
Primary care and community placements provide a safe learning environment for you to familiarise yourselves with talking to children, their families and understanding parents' concerns. Child health is fascinating but many students may find such subjects intimidating.

Fortunately you can practise talking with children and their parents during general practice sessions and at community clinics, such as those for child vaccination. These opportunities, alongside some guidance from your tutors, will show you how to differentiate between what's normal and physiological or pathological. Similarly such clinical exposure reinforces which conditions are common, important for you to know about, as opposed to the much more serious but rarer disease which you are more likely to come across in hospital settings.

Understanding normal child development, how this is monitored and the healthcare professionals involved is a good start. Learning about national vaccination programmes, parental concerns and the public health

TASK

Consider how to assess children and what to think about when an acutely ill child is brought in to be seen. Spend some time with the duty doctor and nurse practitioner, if your practice has one, both of whom will be responsible for triaging and assessing children. Familiarise yourself with national guidelines for assessing unwell children, such as the UK's NICE guidance.

issues associated with such initiatives is also possible. Common childhood illness such as upper respiratory tract infections, earache, tummy ache and diarrhoea and vomiting frequently present in general practice and provides you with opportunities to learn to differentiate between what's self-limiting minor illness and what needs further attention.

Talking to more than one person during a consultation is common during community sessions. Young children obviously bring a carer with them which tends to be a parent, but not always. So try not to make assumptions and always introduce yourself and find out who you are speaking with. Chapter 4 discusses more in detail concerning how best to handle such consultations. Observing how different healthcare professionals speak to children and their carers, handle parental concerns, deal with multiple agendas and sometimes lots of people in the consulting room can be a very useful learning experience for you. Paediatric community attachments are excellent opportunities for you to learn about Safeguarding Children Principles and the practicalities of protecting our most vulnerable patients.

Women's health

Women present more frequently to their doctors, and routine consultations for contraception for example, provide valuable opportunities for healthcare professionals to promote the health of women. Health screening initiatives such as the national cervical screening programme and mammography can be learned about in the community. You will see women who attend for screening and be able to discuss with them their understanding of such initiatives.

TASK

Consider the epidemiology of coronary artery disease in women compared with men and discuss why it may be that diagnosis and investigation of such disease in women may be delayed?

Women present more commonly with issues concerned with mental health and general practice gives you lot of opportunities to learn about how to manage patient's symptoms of anxiety, depression, alcohol excess and less commonly issues pertaining to domestic violence.

Women's health concerns more than just gynaecology, though general practice presents excellent opportunities for you to learn about contraception, menstrual problems and pregnancy and unwanted pregnancy. Women's health raises awareness of not treating women as men in terms of diagnosing illness and also prescribing medicines. Some conditions are more common in women, for example, gallbladder disease, and some drugs are metabolised differently, requiring care on deciding dosage.

Men's health

Men similarly have specific health-related issues that present in the community. Health screening for hypertension and other risk factors associated with an increased risk of heart attack and stroke are important aspects of male health promotion. Patient concerns with testicular self-examination, erectile dysfunction and prostate disease screening are common GP presentations. Excessive alcohol consumption and smoking are issues that affect men's health and can be addressed effectively within primary care.

Looking after older people

Many patients, seen by their GPs, are elderly and these patients give students a good insight into how older people manage their health, cope with their symptoms and deal with their disabilities. There are

---

TASK: LEARNING ABOUT COMPLEX PATIENTS

Ask your GP tutor to identify an elderly patient with several long-term conditions. Meet and interview the patient with a focus on these specific areas:
- Think about all the needs the patient has. Which of these are being met well and which are not?
- What are the patient's priorities? What do they see as essential to be able to do in life? Are these priorities the same as those the doctor and primary health care team (PHCT) focus on?
- Who is involved in their care? How often do they see those people?
- What challenges are there for patients with several long-term conditions? Discuss the patient's care with your tutor.
  Start by telling the patient's story in a narrative style.
  What challenges for the patient have you identified, and what thoughts have you to make care more effective for this patient?

more than three million people aged over 80 living in the United Kingdom, and this number is expected to almost double by 2030 (Kings Fund, 2012). More than 37 million people in the United States, born before 1964 (60% of the population), will have more than one long-term condition by 2030 (American Hospital Association, 2007). Older adults are increasingly at risk of developing long-term conditions, and by the age of 75 a majority of patients will have two more such conditions (often many more). This presents great challenges when managing and organising their care, and with attendant polypharmacy.

In the United States, 1 out of 3 adults aged 65 years or older fall each year, and falls are the leading cause of injury-related death for this age group. Gaining a better understanding of what a patient requires to remain safely at home, including what support their carers require, is important for you as students to grasp so that you can safely discharge patients from hospital when the time comes and engage effectively in planning their on-going care which will be primarily community based.

Many of our elderly patients are both on a variety of and multiple medications. Any drug review of an elderly patient provides ample opportunities for you to learn or revise pharmacological treatments for common conditions, such as hypertension and diabetes. The care of elderly patients presents opportunities to learn about how GPs are responsible for integrating the provision of care for these patients that frequently involves multiple agencies and multidisciplinary healthcare professionals.

TASK

Take a look at the Centre for Disease Control and Prevention (CDC) Healthy Aging website (http://www.cdc.gov/aging/)

This website provides an enormous amount of information about helping elderly Americans lead healthy enjoyable lives, much of which is directly applicable to many other international contexts.

Mental health

A variety of common conditions that affect the mental health of our patients are managed within primary care. GPs are trained to screen for and treat, for example, any associated depression that may accompany long-term chronic conditions, such as rheumatoid arthritis. Diagnoses of cancer and terminal illness may also precipitate symptoms of depression and anxiety which require treatment. Primary care therefore presents opportunities to understand not only common mental health conditions but also how they co-exist with other conditions and affect the lives of patients.

Depression and anxiety present in primary care and the associated morbidity of such conditions has been underreported. There are a variety of screening tools that facilitate making such a diagnosis and helping doctors and nurses decide on subsequent management. You should be aware of and familiar with using patient health questionnaires (PHQ-9) and general anxiety disorder (GAD) scores.

Later clinical years

Towards the end of your training you will appreciate time in general practice as it gives you lot of opportunities to practise for final examinations and revise conditions for which you may have had insufficient time or opportunity to study. Additionally the nature of the doctor–patient interaction facilitates learning about and preparing you for your own independent practice. You will have time to now consider the patient and put all that you have learned into practice. Primary care provides opportunities for clinical 'apprentice style' attachments that encourage you to take on more responsibility for the care of patients with appropriate supervision. This means seeing patients on your own, initiating a management plan and following up patients yourself.

> In the final year, students must use practical and clinical skills, rehearsing their eventual responsibilities as an F1 doctor. These must include making recommendations for the prescription of drugs and managing acutely ill patients under the supervision of a qualified doctor
>
> GMC (2009) Tomorrows Doctors Para 109

Now is the time to consider primary care as a specialty and also decide what knowledge and skills you should learn to better understand how, as a junior doctor, you will need to effectively communicate with primary healthcare professionals. This is equally relevant whether your current career preference is general practice or an alternative.

Learning about primary care

Hopefully you would have had several worthwhile attachments in general practice throughout your medical education to date. However a later placement, either before or after final examinations, gives you time to explore general practice as a career option. There are also specific aspects of primary care itself that all students should learn before graduation whether they plan at this stage to become GPs or not. Effective communication, as demonstrated within teams based at a GP surgery and also wider fields such as with district nursing and palliative care teams, is paramount. How GPs communicate with their hospital colleagues in referring patients and the referral process itself is also an essential prerequisite for all junior doctors, so that they can appreciate the context of the many referrals they receive from the community. Similarly, understanding how receiving clear, relevant and helpful written information from hospitals, in the form of legible or electronic patient discharge summaries, can facilitate the effective transfer of a patient's care back to the GP and help prevent further readmission.

Majority of healthcare takes place in the community and medical students need to be aware of how this is organised and the role primary care has in structuring an efficient affordable NHS, both for the present and the future. The cost of medical interventions, treatment and medications are high and general practice can help you to appreciate how to cost-effectively treat your patients without sacrificing the high quality care we all wish to provide. Therefore during your primary care placements relevant audits and time taken to understand local and national care pathways are valuable assets to your learning.

Learning about prescribing and management plans

Many students feel inadequately prepared in prescribing when they first qualify. General practice and community pharmacy attachments staged throughout your curriculum can ensure that you have plenty of both theoretical teaching and practical experience in prescribing. While medical school will provide the basic underpinning pharmacology teaching every clinical encounter within general practice can illustrate a drug or prescribing issue for you to learn about. GP tutors will supervise you practising writing prescriptions, entering the medication onto the electronic patient record and encourage you to review patients' medication. This encourages you as a student to consider the potential drug interactions, side-effects and risks of any additional medication you may think is necessary. We will explore this more fully in Chapter 5.

You will learn about groups of drugs and their uses. We suggest you actively look for patients with the relevant conditions to interview about their medication. These encounters allow you to integrate your knowledge and deepen your understanding about medications, their uses, side effects, interactions and how patients view their medications.

TASK

Many of you will be given a project to do that involves researching a chronic disease and exploring the experience of patients, their carers and how such conditions are managed within the community. This would also involve reviewing local and national guidance on management, prescribing and referral pathways. This also gives you the chance to help the practice that you are attached to by sharing any updates on good practice and reviewing any audits that you may complete as part of your project.

For example, monitoring blood pressure readings of patients treated for hypertension is a common task within general practice. What is the most commonly prescribed antihypertensive in the practice? Does this fit with local and national guidance on prescribing for treating hypertension? If not can you think of some reasons why this may be so?

General practice facilitates students' practical prescribing by encouraging students in their final years to see patients on their own and begin to initiate their management. Perhaps the earlier part of your training concentrated on listening to patients, learning about taking a clinical history and becoming competent at clinical examination, now is the time to really hone your skills at discussing and explaining to patients the issues that are of concern to them and jointly agree a management plan. This will often include prescribing decisions, and also self-care, support, referral and follow-up plans.

All treatment and management decisions will always be fully supervised, but suggesting to a GP tutor what you think should be the next steps in terms of investigation and/or medication and then issuing the prescription and/or laboratory blood forms or imaging for the GP to sign off can be very satisfying. Later year attachments in general practice expect students to be ready to take on the whole process of seeing patients, making a diagnosis and agreeing a management plan.

Learning in the community 'out of hours'

The increasing access to care and services for patients across the world has brought about a change in provision of settings and accessibility. There has been a long history of provision of out-of-hours primary care services in the United Kingdom, delivered by general practitioners and supported by the Accident and Emergency departments at hospital. There is also some evidence that difficulty in accessing in-hours services in English general practice is associated with increased use of out-of-hours primary care services, regardless of age, gender, ethnicity, deprivation, presence of chronic disease and employment status (Zhou *et al.*, 2015).

As students, you should be encouraged and supported to see the delivery of patient management and care. The general practice may be situated in a health centre or polyclinic, your tutor may be a clinician who continues to work in the local emergency or 'out-of-hours' centres. These centres are not commonly visited by students for learning, yet they provide a rich variety of clinical expertise and care to patients. These settings will offer chances to you to learn from a variety of health professionals working there and you come to understand the importance of good interprofessional communication and excellent clinical skills in settings that do not have the full diagnostic service support available in hospital. Senior students will need to recognise the importance of understanding and managing clinical risk in these situations. Attendance at these clinical settings and discussion with tutors will develop these skills.

Acute medical conditions in both adults and children are generally seen more often than surgical conditions in both out-of-hours and walk-in centres. Skills in identifying accurately the acutely ill patient are needed to avoid missed or delayed diagnoses. The ability to 'read' unusual signs or symptoms is crucial, together with an empathic approach to a consultation that is unsupported by prior knowledge of the patient or their past records. Additionally, you need to recognise that a healthy level of suspicion for the unusual is an important clinical skill, especially when seeing non-indigent individuals. This is not always easy — you need to develop the skills to recognise the symptom or sign that doesn't fit; that comes from experience.

> This experience supplemented my SSC in Emergency Medicine that I did previously in the year. It was in my GP out of hours session that I saw patients being triaged. This will be useful for my FY2 jobs in A + E and general practice, but I don't think it will directly help me in my FY1 jobs – except perhaps to give me an appreciation of the route of the patient from presentation to ward admission
>
> Medical student attending out of hours centre; sourced from O'Brien (2011).

TASK: LEARNING IN OUT-OF-HOURS SETTINGS

As a final year student ask your tutor to arrange a session in an 'out-of-hours' centre. Shadow the doctor or advanced nurse practitioners on duty to experience the challenges involved.

Consider the quality of experience for both the patient and the clinical staff. Explore patients' reasons for the choice of healthcare site.

Consider the areas of clinical and personal risk when consulting in out-of-hours settings. What approaches might reduce those risks?

Explore with your practice tutor the patients seen out-of-hours (electronic notifications are sent in daily). Discuss issues raised with your tutor and peers.

Further opportunities

Selected student components and electives

Most medical schools offer student selected components (SSCs) as part of each year's curriculum. These will give you opportunities to experience aspects of medicine outside of the core curriculum. SSCs may run over a period of only a few weeks or may be integrated into the week. Electives usually provide a longer independent period of study, with many UK students choosing to go overseas. Many students from outside the United Kingdom choose to come and experience British general practice.

Many GPs have specialist interests alongside maintaining their core GP roles which can interest students. GPs with a special interest (called GPwSI in the United Kingdom) have undergone further specialist training and often wish to use this knowledge showing students how general practice and hospital specialties can work together to optimise the care of patients. Attachments in community-orientated ophthal-mology, dermatology and other minor specialties can provide useful SSCs for you when your main curriculum is often so full that you have limited time to follow either interests of your own or areas which you feel have been neglected. GPs may work in areas of social deprivation and be responsible for specific drug, alcohol and rehabilitation programmes, caring for the health needs of the homeless, refugees and/ or people who have been subjected to torture.

As medical students, you may wish to spend more time in primary care than your core curriculum allows. Selecting to spend your elective in gen-eral practice, either abroad or in the United Kingdom, will give you opportunities to explore what primary care and community provision provides for patients. You can, for example, compare how general practice works in different geographical areas, comparing practices between urban and rural settings. The comparison may be eye-opening, and help you decide whether you wish to practice in either of these settings.

Rural, remote health and other interesting placements

Providing primary care services in remote and rural areas is challeng-ing. The pattern of disease is different from urban areas; and, because of the distances from hospital, the range of services provided also tends to be wider. Rural practitioners often provide emergency care, and in some remote areas they may have to manage critically sick or injured patients for a number of hours before these patients can be transferred. To allow patients to remain near their family and to avoid long and ardu-ous journeys there is a need for home or community-based services, such as palliative care or rehabilitation. Many remote and rural areas have community hospitals, and in some areas GPs run acute hospitals that provide emergency and inpatient care with remote tertiary support (MacVicar et al., 2012).

In the UK setting such rural placements will be seen mainly in parts of Northern England, Wales and Scotland. More dramatic examples of remote practice are seen in Canada, Australia and New Zealand and other more sparsely populated countries. You should try to spend some time in a rural clinical setting in order to experience this very different approach to community-based care. If you are not in a medical school with such placements available, consider arranging student selected time or an elective placement in such a setting.

While for some of you a placement in a remote or rural setting may be something new and exciting, others may wish to explore other aspects of primary care medicine or general practice. The beauty of it is the variety, both for students' experiences and as a career. Explore the options available with your medical school and use your time and elective opportunities wisely. A list of interesting placements would include prison medicine, working with refugees and asylum seekers, primary care for the homeless or other hard to reach groups and of course a whole range of options in less developed countries.

Audits and research projects

Many undergraduate curricula require students to undertake research projects, and all of them stipulate that students need to understand the principles underpinning good research and audit. General practice and community attachments expose you to a wide range of topics and the necessary support for you to engage in both audit and research projects across the curriculum. There are ample opportunities for you to take part in simple audits in your early years and sometimes these audits form part of your assessments. Audit helps us understand how data about patients, stored in general practice, can be analysed to show how care can be improved and facilitate the review of typical daily activities such as variance in referral rates. Many practices will expect you to present your findings and consider how best to disseminate any significant outcomes. The development of practice leaflets, posters and patient information sheets by students are common.

Conducting research while on community attachments will facilitate your overall understanding of the field, help you think about career choices, improve your academic skills and contribute to your CV. While not all of you will have the time to take on a research project, it is expected that you will read around the main areas of controversy in practising in general practice and critically appraise some of the relevant leading research articles to ensure your knowledge is up to date.

The costs of healthcare are escalating globally. In many countries the cost of treatments and new medical procedures is spiralling out of control. Common clinical pathways have been introduced into general practice to facilitate efficiencies and cost-effectiveness in many countries within Europe such as, the United Kingdom, Belgium and Holland (www.e-p-a.org). Understanding the underlying research and scientific principles that help design some of these pathways may be an area for your own study and research.

TASK

For example, how valid is some of the clinical pathway guidance? Why not have a look at some of the empirical evidence that helped produce a clinical pathway that is relevant to your community attachment and consider how it lead to its design and how you might explore its implementation within the practice.

Summary

This chapter has covered a wide range of content that you may learn about in general practice and community settings. Emphasis has been placed on how early attachments lay the foundations for later clinical placements, how community placements complement both your science and hospital teaching, and highlights specific elements of the syllabus that you can only learn about when in the community.

While this first chapter has concentrated on what you should and will learn, it has also introduced ideas about how best to learn, which approaches you may find helpful, and how the book as a whole can support and encourage you to make the most of your community learning opportunities.

The following chapters therefore explore these areas in more depth, with Chapter 3 describing about the necessary preparations to make before beginning a community attachment, and then providing plenty of practical advice.

References

American Hospital Association; First Consulting Group (2007) When I'm 64: how boomers will change health care. Chicago: American Hospital Association, 23 p.

Barker R (2010) The future of medicine—avoiding a medical meltdown. New York: Oxford University Press.

Boenink AD, Oderwald AK, de Jonge P, van Tilburg W and Smal JA (2004) Assessing student reflection in medical practice. Medical Education, 38: 368–377.

Dahle LO, Brynhildsen J, Fallsberg MB, Rundquist I and Hammar M (2002) Pros and cons of vertical integration between clinical medicine and basic science within a problem-based undergraduate medical curriculum: examples and experiences from Linkoping, Sweden. Medical Teacher, 24 (3): 280–285.

Dornan T and Bundy C (2004) What can experience add to early medical education? Consensus survey. BMJ, 329 (7470): 834.

GMC (2009) Tomorrows Doctors – Outcomes and Standards for Undergraduate Medical Education. http://www.gmc-uk.org/education/undergraduate/tomorrows_doctors.asp. Accessed 28 March 2014.

Helman CG (2007) Culture, health and illness, 5th Edition. London: Hodder Arnold.

Hilton S (2004) Medical professionalism: how can we encourage it in our students? The Clinical Teacher, 1: 69–73.

MacVicar R, Siderfin C, Williams C and Douglas J (2012) Training the rural GPs of the future. BMJ Careers. Available at http://careers.bmj.com/careers/advice/view-article.html?id=20006803. Morrison, J Medical Education 2006; 40: 495–497.

O'Brien A (2011) Clinical Risk in Unsupported Healthcare Settings: A Pilot Study of Undergraduate Medical Students' Perceptions of placements in Out-of-Hours and Walk-in Centres. Dissertation.

Ogur B and Hirsh D (2009) Learning through longitudinal patient care-narratives from the Harvard Medical School–Cambridge Integrated Clerkship. Academic Medicine, 84: 844–850.

The Kings Fund (2012) The care of frail older people with complex needs: time for a revolution. London: Kings Fund.

World Health Organisation (2002) The World health report 2002: reducing risks, promoting healthy life. Geneva: World Health Organisation.

Zhou Y, Abel G, Warren F, Roland J, Campbell J and Lyratzopoulos G (2015) Do difficulties in accessing in-hours primary care predict higher use of out-of-hours GP services? Evidence from an English National Patient Survey. Emergency Medicine Journal, 32 (5): 373–378.

Further resources

CanMEDS Framework. http://www.royalcollege.ca/portal/page/portal/rc/canmeds/framework. Accessed 29 January 2015.

GMC/Joint Colleges position statement on medical professionalism. http://www.gmc-uk.org/education/undergraduate/professional_behaviour.asp. Accessed 23 June 2015.

Hilton SR and Slotnick HB (2005) Proto-professionalism: how professionalisation occurs across the continuum of medical education. Medical Education 39: 58–65.

Root, trunk and branch model of the determinants of Health Promotion. http://www.healthscotland.com/documents/443.aspx. Accessed 23 June 2015.

Scottish Doctor. www.scottishdoctor.org/. Accessed 23 June 2015.

UN Millennium declaration (2005) http://www.un.org/millenniumgoals/. Accessed 23 June 2015.

Chapter 2 **Learning the public health aspects of medicine**

With Ann O'Brien

One of the great potential strengths of primary care and community health placements is the opportunity to learn about public health. You will have opportunities to do this in all aspects of your placements, from practice-based individual patient contacts (e.g. immunisation and disease screening) to time spent with community and public health specialists planning wider health campaigns or supporting health promotion schemes. In reality, such work is closely integrated with that of day-to-day patient care, and indeed 'learning clinical medicine' – but we have separated the chapters for clarity.

By the end of this chapter you should be able to:

- understand what public health is and its underpinning principles as demonstrated by your community placements
- appreciate how people's health and well-being may be improved by a variety of public health initiatives including health promotion
- understand the role of community screening in reducing ill health and disease
- engage with patients in modifying their lifestyles

Public health perspectives

Medical graduates should be able to: apply to medical practice the principles, method and knowledge of population health and the improvement of health and healthcare.

GMC (2009) Tomorrow's doctors, Outcome 11, p. 17

How to Succeed on Primary Care and Community Placements, First Edition.
David Pearson and Sandra Nicholson.
© 2016 John Wiley & Sons, Ltd. Published 2016 by John Wiley & Sons, Ltd.

What is it that you need to know about public health? Many medical students do not understand the relevance of public health topics and to be fair, sometimes the subject is poorly integrated into medical curricula, failing to highlight what it is that you do need to know at your level. One of the most important issues for students to grasp is how socioeconomic factors are closely related to patients' health and their experience of illness worldwide. Primary care focuses on individual patients and their problems, but public health colleagues remind us of those past significant medical advances such as the eradication of small pox through vaccination, or the reduction of cholera by implementing good sanitation, and encourage you to examine more widely the issues that make people ill, and just as importantly how you can help change things. This remains true today; poor housing, poor education, poor diet and poor lifestyle choices increase the risks of premature death and disability. Public health changes will always make more difference to people's overall health than the expertise of individual clinicians. Globally the situation is stark – with poverty, war, climate change, famine, disease epidemics and the displacements of people impacting significantly on their health. Many undergraduate curricula include topics that highlight such global health issues but there is also much to learn concerning public health embedded in your local communities.

Your community placements in the early years of your course can highlight how public health issues impact upon patients' lives. Such experiences not only reinforce the theoretical perspectives delivered by your medical school teaching but also provide memorable, and sometimes inspirational, encounters with patients or community leaders. You will see public health interventions in action – flu vaccinations and cervical

TASK

On your placement explore interventions or local projects which help identify and ameliorate the effects of poverty on health.

Public health issues are often stipulated learning objectives assessed by case studies or log book entries.

Ask your tutor to help you find patients who you can talk to and sensitively explore how their housing or environment affects their health, and how the practice you are attached to supports public health initiatives.

screening are examples, but also more personal public health issues such as patient requests for help with social housing applications.

Primary care is the setting for a significant delivery of public health matters and gives you the opportunity to see the practical relevance of this important topic. The role of primary care health professionals as advocates for health promotion and health education for chronic disease or illness prevention is important but these areas are broad and not necessarily fully implemented. The use of the UK's Quality Outcomes Framework (http://www.hscic.gov.uk/qof) in general practice is an opportunity for high quality evidence-based teaching at the community–individual interface. You need to ensure you have discussions with your tutors and peers about topics identified from your curriculum that are important from a population-based health perspective.

There are many factors that influence public health over the course of a patient's lifetime. They all need to be understood and acted upon and, a community setting provides ample experiences for you to learn about these issues. In recent years, plans have progressed to integrate public health into local government so that local health services for patients will be planned and delivered in the context of the broader social

---

TASK: A PUBLIC HEALTH PROJECT

With your peers on placement take time to read and reflect upon a recent UK Department of Health framework which focuses on the two high-level outcomes to be achieved across the UK public health system and beyond:

1 Increased healthy life expectancy
2 Reduced differences in life expectancy between communities

These outcomes will be delivered through improvements across a range of public health indicators, grouped into four domains relating to the three pillars of public health: health protection, health improvement and healthcare public health; as well as improving the wider determinants of health (Dept Health, 2013).

- As a group of students, share the sections of this document and think how these issues affect people's lives and health.
- Meet as a group to discuss what you have found and how it applies to the patients you are currently seeing.

determinants of health, like poverty, education, housing, employment, crime and pollution. The NHS, social care, the voluntary sector and communities will all work together to make this happen.

Health promotion

Health promotion has been defined by the World Health Organization as:

> ...The process of enabling people to increase control over their health and its determinants, and thereby improve their health. It is a core function of public health and contributes to the work of tackling communicable and non-communicable diseases and other threats to health
>
> WHO (2005)

Public health and health promotion create an agenda that moves beyond the focus on individual behaviour towards a wide range of social and environmental interventions. Health promotion strategies are neither limited to a specific health problem, nor to a specific set of behaviours. The World Health Organization applies the principles of and strategies for health promotion to a variety of population groups, risk factors, diseases and in various settings. Health promotion, and the associated efforts put into education, community development, policy, legislation and regulation, is equally valid for prevention of communicable diseases, injury and violence and mental problems, as they are for prevention of non-communicable diseases (WHO, 2013).

You will have a chance in community settings to understand what is meant by health promotion, and how healthcare professionals engage with patients to encourage healthy lifestyles and prevent disease. You will learn what part health promotion plays in the doctor–patient consultation and that of other healthcare professionals. There will be opportunities to explore the risk factors associated with common chronic medical conditions and consider how best to advise patients about reducing their risk. General practice is an ideal setting in which you understand how many conditions are exacerbated by a culmination of risk factors which work together to increase a patient's individual risk of illness and/or complications. A vital part of a doctor's remit is to help prevent disease and educate patients about how to stay healthy. The health costs associated with maintaining healthcare services and providing expensive treatments are spiralling in all countries. Primary care provides you with opportunities to participate in providing inexpensive treatments designed to prevent diseases from occurring, for example, smoking cessation clinics.

TASK

Identify a health promotion intervention within the practice or placement, for example, posters or visual presentations, smoking cessation clinics, walking clubs, slimming clinics, exercise classes.
- What risk factors is the intervention aiming to reduce?
- Research the relevant epidemiology of the condition and its risk factors.
- How effective do you think such a health promotion intervention may be?
- What evidence is there to justify your conclusions?

Primary and secondary disease prevention

An important part of public health work is the organisation of primary and secondary screening in order to identify serious illnesses early on (and ideally treat or ameliorate its progression). Screening for ill-health and long-term conditions are a key part of the everyday work for both GPs and the primary health care team. You will see clearly during your community placements where the overlaps with and tensions between national health programmes and individual health concerns occur.

Screening for cancer and long-term conditions are organised nationally but implemented locally, usually through primary care and community services. The most well-known UK programmes include the national cervical cancer screening programme, the breast screening programme and recently the faecal occult blood screening for colon cancer. You will have the chance to discuss these initiatives with clinicians and patients, and consider their effectiveness in the light of the principles of good screening. Health professionals in primary care spend a considerable time either encouraging people to enter appropriate screening programmes or often explaining concerns when results are not reassuring.

TASK

Undertake an audit of uptake of cervical screening in your placement.
Compare your results with that of the National figures.
Discuss the implications of the results.
Explore with patients reasons for lack of uptake of screening invitations.

Primary health care teams, and specifically general practitioners in the United Kingdom, are all involved with the early identification of patients with impaired glucose tolerance, diabetes, renal disease and of course ischaemic heart disease. Approaches to identification include opportunistic and systematic methods, and case finding using bloods tests and risk tools. Risk tools are being increasingly used to establish cardiovascular risk, and this provides rich opportunities for your learning, both about these important approaches and the conditions themselves.

The UK's Quality Outcome Framework [QoF] is a core part of the General Medical Services (GMS) contract for general practices and offers a framework of national quality standards for long-term conditions based on the best available, research-based evidence. We have included an example, but this framework is annually updated and you should access the link for the latest information (http://www.hscic.gov.uk/qof). This framework, and its equivalents in other countries, should offer a valuable framework to your own learning, helping prioritise and structure your clinical learning as well as reinforce how public health policy can be made effective for individual patients via consultations in primary care. The subsequent task provides further direction about how the QoF can help you plan your learning.

Examples of QoF: Clinical indicators (*Example only – see text above*)

| AF002 | The percentage of patients with atrial fibrillation in whom stroke risk has been assessed using the CHADS2 risk stratification scoring system in the preceding 2 months (excluding those whose previous CHADS2 score is greater than 1) |
| CHD006 | The percentage of patients with a history of myocardial infarction (on or after 1 April 2011) currently treated with an ACE-I (or ARB if ACE-I intolerant), aspirin or an alternative anti-platelet therapy, beta-blocker and statin |

HYP004	The percentage of patients with hypertension aged 16 or over and who have not attained the age of 75 in whom there is an assessment of physical activity, using GPPAQ, in the preceding 12 months
DM014	The percentage of patients newly diagnosed with diabetes, on the register, in the preceding 1 April to 31 March who have a record of being referred to a structured education programme within 9 months after entry on to the diabetes register

TASK

Ask your tutor or practice manager to familiarise you with the various domains in QoF or your equivalent national guideline.
- What other disease areas have clinical indicators in QoF?
- What health promotion and prevention indicators are there?
- Discuss one domain (relevant to your current learning) with your tutor and peers.
- How do the indicators affect individual care?
- What are the benefits and concerns at individual and population level?

This then needs to lead to discussions about modification of risk factors. Explanation of the risk–benefit of lifestyle modifications is a difficult consultation; we will look in the next section about how you can learn those skills during your placements.

TASK

Request to see the online database to explore the outcomes for the QoF (or national equivalent) for your local surgery.
- How do the practice figures compare against others in the local area and then nationally?
- Having understood these variations, discuss with your tutor and peers what factors may be impacting on any differences observed.

Behaviour change: health promotion and prevention for individuals

Advice to patients includes all topics that will support patients to make lifestyle changes for their health benefit. Smoking cessation is the most commonly known activity; specific training for practice nurses allows this to be delivered in primary care. The ability to observe motivational interviewing or health coaching techniques will provide a useful skill for you to learn about behaviour change. The cycle of change is widely used where changes in health behaviour is required. It describes five stages of readiness and provides a framework for understanding the change process (Prochaska and DiClemente, 1982). It allows interventions to be tailored to the individual's 'readiness' to progress in the recovery process.

Patients with cardiovascular disease, diabetes and obesity will be encouraged to address lifestyle behaviours that impact their conditions. Specialised referral schemes for exercise and dietary advice are available in the community. The engagement of patients and mechanisms required to make suitable changes can be observed when on placement. You may also observe lifestyle and behaviour change being discussed by local drug and alcohol units, sexual health professionals and many others. Try to engage closely with these opportunities – ideally as an active participant. This means thinking about, discussing with your tutor and planning how such consultations should be structured to allow you to get the maximum learning opportunities. Initially observing the interactions between patients and healthcare professionals should progress to starting to discuss with patients themselves about their lifestyles and possible health promotion initiatives. You should also reflect on what you have seen that appears to be more effective in bringing about change.

TASK

Explore with your tutor opportunities to observe and support behaviour change for health benefits. This may involve working with dieticians, practice nurses, drug and alcohol workers or specialist nurses (e.g. diabetes or cardiovascular team).
- Identify where patients are on the cycle of change?
- What interventions can be used to encourage commitment?
- How effective are these interventions?

Public health and health education

In a context of growing inequity, competition for scarce natural resources and a financial crisis threatening basic entitlements to health care, it would be hard to find a better expression of health as a fundamental right, as a prerequisite for peace and security, equity, social justice, popular participation and global solidarity...

WHO Twelfth General Programme of Work (GPW12)

The public health of world countries is impacted by climate change, migration, changing population demographics, unemployment, technology, rapid urbanisation and economic fluctuations leading to changes in health funding. As a world society we need to consider what personal responsibilities we have for trying to meet the fundamental right of health (http://www.who.int/about/resources_planning/WHO_GPW12_setting_the_scene.pdf).

Public Health England was established in 2013 to protect and improve the health and well-being of patients and to reduce inequalities. It follows the development of a 21st-century health and well-being service, supporting local authorities and the NHS to deliver improvements in public health. The UK's National Institute for Clinical Excellence (NICE) has produced guidelines that focus on the public health needs of populations and approaches to disease prevention and patient well-being (http://www.nice.org.uk/About/What-we-do/Our-Programmes/NICE-guidance/NICE-guidelines/NICE-public-health-guidelines). They cover mental health and behavioural conditions, endocrine diseases, nutritional and metabolic conditions, digestive system disorders, infectious diseases and cardiovascular diseases. Approaches to the interventions in these areas include behavioural change, diet management, increased activity and working with communities. Similar guidelines are produced by many other countries, for example, SIGN (Scotland).

TASK

- Discover any public health initiatives that have taken place in your placement area.
- Discuss with your tutor what was involved and who the target audience was.
- How might you initiate discussions about a new approach to a chronic problem?
- Identify any national guidance, for example, NICE or SIGN, related to the area identified.
- Consider what initiatives might be employed to successfully deliver the public health guidance in the local area, and how does the practice team support these initiatives?

Summary

All doctors have a responsibility to contribute to public health and this chapter has highlighted what this means for you as medical students and how you can begin to engage with public health. The prevention of ill-health and promotion of well-being should be at the forefront of all we do in our professional lives. We have indicated how community health placements highlight the importance of the balance between preventive and curative medical interventions, and how your tutor and his/her colleagues in the primary healthcare team are at the forefront of health promotion and the interface of individual and population medicine. This interface presents opportunities for you to learn about the tensions surrounding the costs of treatment and ethical issues where individual wants and needs have to be balanced with national priorities. Points of tension and debate are good places to learn – engage with it, think about the issues and discuss them with your peers and tutors.

References

Dept Health (2013) Part 1A: A Public Health Outcomes Framework for England, 2013–2016. Available at https://www.gov.uk/government/uploads/system/uploads/attachment_data/file/263658/2901502_PHOF_Improving_Outcomes_PT1A_v1_1.pdf. Accessed 15 July 2015.

GMC (2009) Tomorrows Doctors – Outcomes and Standards for Undergraduate Medical Education. Available at http://www.gmc-uk.org/education/undergraduate/tomorrows_doctors.asp. Accessed 28 March 2014.

NICE Guidelines. http://www.nice.org.uk/About/What-we-do/Our-Programmes/NICE-guidance/NICE-guidelines/NICE-public-health-guidelines. Accessed 21 June 2015.

Prochaska, J.O. & DiClemente, C.C. (1982) Transtheoretical therapy: Toward a more integrative model of change. Pscychotherapy: theory, research and practice, 19, 276–288.

WHO (2005) WHO 6th Global Conference on Health Promotion, Bangkok, Thailand, August 2005.

WHO (2013) Development of a Framework to Promote Action Across Sectors of Health and Health Equity. http://www.who.int/healthpromotion/en/index.html. Accessed February 2014.

WHO (2014) Twelfth General Programme of Work 2014–2019. Available at: http://www.who.int/about/resources_planning/WHO_GPW12_setting_the_scene.pdf. Accessed March 2014.

Chapter 3 **Preparing for and learning on primary care and community placements**

With Maria Hayfron-Benjamin

Introduction

The aim of this chapter is to help you prepare for your community placement. Finding your placement, arriving on time and knowing what you can and need to learn while you are there will help you get a good start. Understanding the practical steps you need to take before going on community placements and some of the principles that contribute to how you learn best within a community setting will help you make the most of them.

We also provide you with guidance on optimising your experience while on your placement. The previous chapters highlighted what you should consider learning and this chapter helps you think about how best to go about this. Students sometimes complain that they don't know what to expect on a placement, or don't know how/what tutors have been asked to prepare for them. This chapter helps you to consider how best to engage your tutors in your learning and how you can learn from your peers and patients. Later chapters go into more detail with specific examples of how to learn from patients and members of primary healthcare team. Finally thinking about what a tutor needs to do to prepare for your placement will also help you better understand what is available and expected of you; you will then be able to give your tutor better feedback on your experience.

How to Succeed on Primary Care and Community Placements, First Edition.
David Pearson and Sandra Nicholson.
© 2016 John Wiley & Sons, Ltd. Published 2016 by John Wiley & Sons, Ltd.

Therefore this chapter is broadly divided into three sections that consider what you need to do ahead of your placement, during your placement and at the end of your placement.

By the end of this chapter you should be able to:

- know how best to prepare for attending your placements
- have some very practical tips to guide your learning while on placement
- understand what is expected of you following your placement

Arrival at medical school is an exciting time; the culmination, for most of you, of years of preparation, studying, undertaking work experience, soul searching, researching career options, pros and cons of different medical schools. While you will appreciate the need to learn the basic science underpinning your future practice, you will also be desperately keen to see real doctors looking after real patients in clinical settings. As a new medical student you will also want to see patients for yourself. Attachments in primary care and the community provide the opportunities to do this from the very beginning of your training and all the way through.

A clinical placement can be defined as 'Any arrangement in which a medical student is present in an environment that provides healthcare or related services to patients and the public. Placements can take place in primary, secondary or community healthcare or social care settings' (GMC, 2011). Hence you will gain experiences that enhance your learning across a number and variety of placements and not just general practice. However the preparation and many of the general principles that ensure you get the most out of these placements are the same. You should receive an introduction to the placement ensuring you know what to bring, where to go and what to expect.

Do ensure that you go to all clinical placements with an open mind so you can make the best of any learning opportunity. Following your briefing try to extend your personal knowledge about your placement and its work before attending. Think about your overall course objectives and what resources you may need to accomplish this, for example, books, paper or electronic gadgets.

Most medical schools will send students to a variety of primary care and community settings during your time with them but all medical schools will send students to general practices. Most general practices are small- or medium-sized organisations, therefore unlike a hospital where you may not see familiar faces when you return a week later, in general practice you are much more likely to get to know the practice team, particularly if you are attending on a block or longitudinal placement. General practice offers a number of features that makes it suitable for clinical teaching. The nature of the organisation means that a General Practice will be able to adjust the workload of your tutor because they are teaching, that is, they may have teaching time scheduled into their day and may not be seeing patients while they are teaching you, or set specific time aside for tutorials so you get some focussed teaching. This is in addition to the arrangements that attachments have made to ensure that your clinical exposure is appropriate and maximised.

The clue is in the name: in general practice you will see a variety of patients and presentations, but at the same time all practices will have some patients that are relevant to your current learning needs. Therefore, whatever you are there to learn about, it should be possible for you to see relevant patients, for example, if you are on placement for a day and learning about diabetes, every practice will have patients with type 1 and type 2 diabetes, they will have patients whose diabetes is well controlled, newly diagnosed patients, expert patients, patients that have been found to be at risk of developing diabetes. So even if your placement day does not coincide with a diabetes clinic, it should be possible for your tutors to invite relevant patients to meet you or to arrange for you to visit patients at home. This means your tutor will go to a great length to ensure that you get the appropriate opportunity to see patients and learn what you need to know. It is therefore vital for you to prepare for these placements. This chapter will help you think what you will need to do.

For most students learning in a clinical environment will be a new way of learning. In most classroom-based teaching meeting the learning needs of the students is the focus, whereas in a clinical environment, service delivery and meeting the needs of patients is the focus. Whilst meeting the learning needs of students is important this is secondary to addressing patients' healthcare needs. In addition you will encounter a variety of different environments – out-patient clinics, patients' homes, day-centres, schools, hospital wards, general practices. Tutors will have varying teaching styles; you may be on placement with students from other professional groups or medical students who are senior or more junior to you. In short, learning in clinical settings can be messy.

Preparing for your community placements

How to get there

To get the most from your placement it pays to do some preparatory work. To begin with, find out how to get there, sometimes you may be given detailed instructions and travel advice, or you may simply be given a name, the postal and/or e-mail address of your tutor. Even if you have been given travel advice it is worth checking if that applies from where you live. There are a number of websites that you can use to plan your journey; for example, in London the Transport for London website (http://journeyplanner.tfl.gov.uk) is comprehensive.

If possible think about travelling with another student or car pooling where necessary. Do allow extra time on the first morning or do a trial run. It is not conducive to your learning if you arrive late and flustered and it will not help your tutors or colleagues either. Attachments will conduct an induction, provide a timetable, introduce members of the team to you, and show you around the premises on arrival – all very

---

TIPS: BEING WELL PREPARED FOR YOUR PLACEMENT

- Plan your journey in advance, have a back-up plan in case of problems.
- Ensure you have the name of the tutor, the address and the telephone number of the placement with you in case you encounter unexpected difficulties, if possible keep contact details of fellow students on placement with you.
- Don't waste travel time! Use the time on the train or the bus to flick through the British National Formulary or Oxford Handbook of Clinical Medicine.
- Find out about the area before you get there – the more you know about the patients and conditions, the better you will be able to engage fully with the opportunities the placement offers.
- Do any preparatory work that has been set for you.

helpful and not to be missed. This is a further opportunity for you to demonstrate your professionalism and commitment to medicine.

Health and safety on community placements

The vast majority of student–patient encounters in clinical settings occur without incident. Histories are taken, patients are examined, and supervised procedures done, students learn and patients go away often happy to have helped a new 'doctor'. However, things can go wrong and in a worst case scenario your action or omission might cause harm to the patient either because you made a mistake or you were not properly trained or supervised. Sometimes your words or actions might be misinterpreted by a patient or a relative leading to a complaint or an allegation of an abuse. It is important that you and the patient are adequately protected. One essential protection is insurance in case something goes wrong.

The various ways in which medical students are indemnified are complex and may be subject to change. It depends on whether they are on medical school premises; state health premises, for example, a hospital or community clinic; or on private property, for example, in a GP surgery or in a patient's home. Your medical school will be able to provide you with more specific and up-to-date information about local policies. In the United Kingdom, the General Medical Council (GMC, 2011) sets out its expectations and the arrangements that it wants to see in place for medical students relating to indemnity. It's important you find out before your placement starts what is required of you and that your school has explained its arrangements to you.

During your time at medical school there will be opportunities for you to meet representatives from a range of professional organisations and associations in addition to the clubs and societies that you may want to join. It is worth investing some time speaking to those representatives to find out what they offer and how they might be able to help you, for example, some will offer free membership to medical students. Our advice to you is to be mindful of your own and your patient's safety in clinical settings. Always ensure you are fully supervised, and that you take up membership of one of the medical defence organisations before you start any clinical placement including any occasional visits to clinical settings in the early years.

When you arrive on placements

Please remember all clinical placements are working environments where service delivery is the primary concern, sometimes patients refuse to see students, or feel too unwell to participate in teaching. You may have days where your patient contact is less than you might hope for. At the end of your clinical placement you will be asked to provide some feedback for your tutors. This will be discussed in more detail at the end of this chapter but for now remember that your feedback should be constructive and specific.

Your tutors have been busy preparing for your arrival, and following are some reasonable expectations that you should have of them:

- someone is designated as the point of contact and is responsible for continuity for you – this should normally include a named administrator who deals with 'teaching' and a named clinical tutor responsible for your education while in the community or practice placement;
- tutors should provide clear instructions on what students should do if they are unwell or running late, that is, who should they contact – tutor, reception, administrator; how should they make contact – mobile phone, telephone, e-mail;
- that the practice and the designated tutors are not over-committed and demonstrate a manageable clinical/teaching balance;
- if they have students from different years, or even different medical schools, your timetable shows a fair proportion of opportunities for you to reach your learning goals;
- a timetable that clearly lays out the opportunities for you to learn not only during the sessions that you are present for, but also builds in

---

TIP

Use any downtime wisely! You will sometimes be asked to wait outside when a patient doesn't want a medical student to hear about their problem, or doesn't want you to be present for an intimate examination. Use this time well, flick through the Oxford Handbook or equivalent and look up disease! Refer the pharmacy handbook, British National Formulary (BNF) or equivalent formulary and look up the relevant drugs that you may have come across that day in the consultation.

some flexibility into the plan for the day/week/unit. This is because you may cover any specific needs, for example, you may have seen lots of cardiac patients in high-dependency settings but may feel under-confident in managing undifferentiated chest pain.

Professionalism on community placements

Being a medical student, particularly while on a clinical placement, puts you in a privileged position. You may find that members of the public, complete strangers will be prepared to/may want to speak to you about their medical problems, they may be prepared to discuss personal information that they may not have shared with their partners/children/ closest friends – all because you have met the entry requirements and been accepted into medical school. Individuals will have expectations of you because they are meeting you in a clinical setting or because you have been introduced to them by someone involved in their healthcare. People do not always distinguish between a student in week 1 of the course and a final-year student. If you happen to be a bit older than some of your peers, you may find that people expect you to be a senior even if you have told them you are in the first year.

As a medical student you are expected to behave 'professionally' from the start of your medical school experience. What do we mean by 'professionally'? Definitions abound – from Cosgrove who defines a professional doctor as one who does 'the right thing, at the right time, for the right reasons' (Cosgrove, 2006) to the more structured definition of professionalism from Eraut (1994) who identifies five component parts:

- a moral commitment to serve the clients' interests;
- the discipline to self-monitor and review personal practice;
- the will to expand one's personal repertoire and reflect on one's experience;
- to contribute to your organisation;
- and to reflect on and contribute to the profession's changing role in society.

There will be many opportunities for you to reflect upon these aspects of medical professionalism as you start and progress along your community attachments, both for yourself and the healthcare professionals working with you. You will notice that the relationships community professionals have with patients may be less formal than what you see in a hospital setting. This reminds us that at the heart of professionalism is the trust that patients put in their doctors and this is expected from you as a medical student from the very beginning of your training. This may be demonstrated by simple measures such as always introducing yourself and explaining who you are and what role you play, wearing your name badge and never attempt to advise or do things with patients that you are not sufficiently trained or confident in doing.

The United Kingdom's GMC in their Good medical practice document sets out the duties of a doctor and provides clear guidance on how doctors should demonstrate their professionalism in each of the four domains:

Domain 1: Knowledge, skills and performance
Domain 2: Safety and quality
Domain 3: Communication, partnership and teamwork
Domain 4: Maintaining trust

GMC, Duties of a Doctor (2013)

As a medical student it is essential that you are aware of these duties and are compliant with them from the start of your medical education. Clearly as a student you will be unable to demonstrate professionalism in all domains as you are not yet in a position to practice independently. However you are expected to be aware of all the aspects and issues and increasingly take on these duties and responsibilities as your experience permits. Community placements provide many opportunities for this, for example, you are required as a student to ensure that any patient you interview or examine has consented to it and sometimes the more informal atmosphere of general practice makes the very formal process of asking patients for consent seem awkward. You will often be out and about visiting patients and travelling between sites, you must keep records containing personal information about patients securely and where possible not take such material off the premises. It's usually possible to anonymise presentations and case histories. There will be opportunities to work collaboratively with peers, other colleagues, and at all times respect the skills and contributions of other disciplines in caring for patients and teaching you. Community placements, particularly those involved with vulnerable patients such as those with mental health issues, drug addiction or simply the frail elderly are opportunities for you to demonstrate that you can treat patients fairly and with respect whatever their life choices and beliefs.

Professional appearance

As an individual you have the right to dress and present yourself as you wish to, however on clinical placements, including community attachments, you will be required to comply with the local dress codes and infection control policies, this may mean, for example, that you should be 'bare below the elbows', that is, no jewellery (except a wedding band) and short or rolled up sleeves, long hair tied up. When meeting patients in a community setting it's important that you should 'Dress in an appropriate and professional way and be aware that patients will respond to your appearance, presentation and hygiene' (GMC, 2009).

Remember that you are not going to an interview, and you will be seeing patients in a community setting including their homes, your clothing should allow you to move freely and should remain in place and not reveal your underwear as you move. In a patient's home you may need to kneel on the floor to examine a leg ulcer, you may have to lean over the patient in their own bed to examine their chest. You should wear appropriate protection when necessary, for example, gloves when examining a wound or collecting a clinical specimen. When you are working with patients there is always a risk that you may become contaminated with bodily secretions, a baby you are examining may urinate on you, or a child with gastroenteritis may vomit when you are examining them. You may find it cost effective to put together a small wardrobe of 'work wear' including smart plain trousers and/or skirts, suitable blouses and shirts, jumpers and cardigans with short or roll-able sleeves that can be easily washed. Always carry your identification and wear your name badge where it can be easily seen.

Practicalities while on placement

Do remember that your community placement may be located in built-up city areas, and that crime can occur anywhere. Some community placements are more remote and isolated than those based in hospitals, which always has lots of people on site. Be aware that your phone/laptop/iPad may put you at risk of being robbed. Keep them out of sight. Do you need to take them with you? Will there be secure storage at the placement? It might be better to print a map/directions to your placement rather than using your phone or tablet to guide you. If you have the appropriate travel pass/ticket in advance you can avoid using your wallet unnecessarily. Where possible travel with colleagues. Seek advice about local safety issues from staff that work there, frequency of buses etc., especially if leaving the placement after dark. Some placements will be in socially deprived areas, and it's important that you have learning opportunities within these areas. However, watch out for each other! If you are leaving the placement base during the daytime, ensure that people know where you are going and when you are expected back. If you are planning to go home directly after a visit to a clinic or a patient's home, make arrangements to text a colleague to let them know that you have done as you planned. Mobile phones are invaluable but need to be used appropriately and safely.

> Take a map or a smart phone! You never know when you'll be on a home visit, so scan the area so you know the main roads! It makes life easier!
>
> (Final-year student)

Ensure you are compliant with any security advice given to you by the staff, for example, not allowing people in restricted areas, wearing your photo ID at all times, taking due care with any keys or security passes issued to you so you can move around the clinical area.

Within this context you need to be aware of other unprofessional dangers of using your mobile phone. Looking up medications and searching for information concerning patients' conditions is entirely appropriate but be careful and ensure that patients and other colleagues are aware of what you are doing when using your phone within a consultation or clinical setting otherwise it could be misconstrued.

It sounds obvious but we remind you to read your placement handbook, your tutors should know what your objectives are for your time with them, however they are humans and may not have memorised all the minor changes in your unit of teaching since they taught it last year. The person that should be most concerned with the tasks that need to be completed on placement is you. If you are required to have three chest examinations and two case presentations signed off in your logbook then this needs to be highlighted at the start of the attachment so that these activities can be factored into your tutor's plan.

TASK

Ask your tutor, if they don't already suggest it, to help you complete a 'learning needs assessment' so that you are aware of your strengths and weaknesses and what you need to focus on during this placement. Think about what you know, don't know and need to know – and what bits you can best learn in the primary care or community placement. Discuss those needs with your tutor as early in the placement as possible.

For any clinical placement there may be specific objectives for each day or there may be an expectation that a number of outcomes are covered throughout your time on placement, additionally there will be assessments that need to be completed while you are on placement and you may have a log book or learning portfolio activities that you need to cover and get signed off. You should check and know what you need to cover before you get to the placement as there may be opportunities to sign off parts of your log book or assessment on day 1.

You should discuss the following with your tutor at the start of your placement:

- how will you be assessed, and do ensure this is discussed early in your placement. Experienced tutors may not have realised that there have been changes, and you may wish to share expectations
- ensure you know what learning outcomes you need to cover on placement
- ensure your tutor knows about any tasks or activities that you need to complete and sign off in addition to your formal assessment, for example, project work, case presentations, etc.
- if you have a portfolio with tasks that need to be signed off ensure you take it with you and that you know what you need to achieve
- your learning needs and what can be realistically achieved while you are on placement
- check that their teaching plan takes your learning needs as well as the course outcomes into consideration.

He is a great teacher and also very friendly and approachable making the whole experience more enjoyable. He involved us well and always asked us about what we wanted to learn, taking our views and interests into consideration as well as working around what the curriculum required.

(Third-year medical student)

Developing personal learning plans and goals

The importance and helpfulness of developing and agreeing with your tutors the learning plans that clarify your aims and objectives to be achieved during your placements has been indicated. Identifying what you know, what you don't know and what you need to know, with the help of your tutor, is probably the best start to any attachment. It sets the scene, indicates the direction for future learning and as Chapter 9 indicates is essential for a rewarding assessment experience.

Your tutors will be interested to help you identify what you personally need to learn, what you consider as yet unmet learning needs as well as covering outlined learning objectives.

> The most important single factor influencing learning is what the learner already knows. Ascertain this and teach him accordingly
>
> (Ausubel *et al.*, 1978)

Therefore an appropriately conducted learning needs analysis with your tutor will help:

- tailor the teaching sessions to meet your needs
- you to understand better your own areas of weakness
- you to develop a capacity for self-assessment.

There are a variety of ways that this can happen. Initially this occurs with your pre-attachment preparation, consideration of the formal learning objectives of the module and through early discussion with your tutors. Tutors may simply discuss with you your experience and confidence of covering stated learning objectives or review any portfolios that you have to complete. Some tutors may use quizzes or simply ask questions to identify areas of weakness. However once on your placement tutor-observed histories, examinations and presenting management plans are ideal opportunities for both of you to agree on what to prioritise. Additional formal information through feedback from patients, peers, staff and other health professionals (e.g. 360° appraisals) is helpful in supplementing your self-assessment of your on-going learning needs. Should you be involved or have the opportunity to listen to any discussion concerning significant incidents or events, you will be able to appreciate how healthcare professionals can learn from these situations (Spencer, 2003).

One of the overall goals of medical education and training is to develop your capability to carry out critical self-reflection of your performance. This will help you become a more effective self-directed and independent professional. Clearly identifying your learning needs plays a key role in helping you develop the skills of critical self-reflection by providing opportunities for self-assessment of your clinical competence, knowledge, understanding and attitudes. With the help of your tutors you can also understand if there exists any mismatch between self-perception and observed behaviour.

One way of doing this is by using Johari's window (adapted from Luff and Ingham, 1950).

	Known to self	Not known to self
Known to others	Open arena	Blind spot
Not known to others	Hidden (façade)	Unknown

Being aware of the issues that Johari's window highlights enables you and your tutor to make the most of the feedback opportunities. Starting a discussion with what you and your tutor think you know and then moving swiftly on to areas that you feel less confident with and highlighting your 'knowledge blind spots' should enable you to gain a good picture of your learning needs for the placement. Discipline yourself to ask 'how do I think that went?' as a means of self-reflection and a chance to review your performance.

You may be seeing different tutors on different days; some may not have seen the assessment criteria at all and hence will be relying on you to keep them informed about what you would like to or what you need to see/do. It can seem daunting to ask/tell your tutors what it is you need to do but the vast majority of tutors take students because they want to help you to become a doctor and many also want you to see how great their specialism is. It will help both of you if you come prepared with realistic and achievable goals for your placement and if you share those with your tutor(s).

Active learning – getting involved

At medical school you will encounter a range of teaching methods; there will be some didactic teaching where an expert teacher delivers a lecture and you sit in a lecture theatre and listen, or watch the podcast later; but a greater proportion of your community time will be spent learning within small groups, in pairs learning with and from each other, and in self-directed independent learning where you, with guidance from your tutors, set your own learning goals. You will also learn a great deal from your tutors who will come from a variety of healthcare backgrounds and disciplines.

When attached to a community setting you may be on your own, in pairs, or in larger groups. Attending a placement in a larger group, say four to six students, provides opportunities for you to work with your peers in groups. Medical schools frequently encourage you to do this as a precursor to clinical team working and as an opportunity for you to learn from each other. Sometimes this will involve shared tasks, presentations and meeting patients together. Alternatively you will each have your own objectives but work alongside each other. Observing how other people work is invaluable and learning how best to work together is indispensable.

> **TASK**
>
> Community placements in pairs provide great opportunities for you to receive and give peer feedback. This should be agreed with your peer in advance and you can plan what areas of feedback you might wish to work on together, for example, if you are doing a patient home visit together, then it is advisable for you to split the history-taking into two, while one is talking with the patient, the other student could make some notes to give to their peer about how effective their communication was or areas to improve upon within the history-taking. You can then swap roles. It would be good to discuss afterwards but take care not to do this in a public place.

It's not always necessary to be the team leader when set to work in teams. Effective team working requires each member to meaningfully contribute. This highlights the equal importance of all the roles people may play within a team. Starter-finishers, that is, those who ensure tasks get finished on time, inspirational members who come up with good ideas but sometimes need the help of others to include sufficient attention to detail, are examples of some of the roles within effective teams.

Frequently your tutor will encourage you to do some preparation before sessions. Revising the underpinning science and basic clinical knowledge required to fully appreciate how to approach patients and learn from their presentations is essential for you to get fully involved.

TASK

Tomorrow you are going to attend the nurse-practitioner run diabetic clinic. What preparation do you think you need to do the night before to get the most out of this session?

Assuming you know about the fundamentals of diabetes (diagnosis, presenting symptoms and typical management) what should you be thinking about in terms of your learning from the clinic? Discuss your ideas with your fellow students so that you get a consensus of what's most important and relevant.

Some suggestions for your preparation might be:
- What are the common complications of long-term diabetes?
- How do healthcare practitioners monitor these?
- What screening occurs at such appointments?

Once present within the clinic you might then specifically observe and ask about:
- How the patient is cared for? What impact does an multidisciplinary team (MDT) have?
- How do the nurse-practitioner and GP work together?
- What do you think are common patient concerns?

Thinking about how best to engage with patients in the community and how to make the most of the opportunities to learn from every patient you meet needs some consideration. Chapter 4 discusses what you can learn from individual interactions between healthcare practitioners and patients. Think about how you can individually learn from patients, how to learn with patients and how to involve patients in your learning. This will encourage you to create a patient-centred focus, which will stand you in good stead for both your learning within the community and subsequently.

Learning to be a doctor

Depending on your level of experience, primary care and community placements will provide varying opportunities for you to learn how to behave as a prospective doctor. You will observe doctor–patient interactions and see how doctors speak to their patients and team members. Starting to talk with patients allows you to begin taking on a professional medical role and as you gain experience, general practice will hone your professional as well as clinical skills. This means that you will begin to understand and be able to act and gain the appropriate attitudes of doctors, albeit in a supervised and initially limited capacity. This type of learning is important. Feeling like a doctor and being treated like one even in a measured manner is very motivational for students and helps you become what you see yourselves as.

Chapter 1 outlined what you can learn when on primary care and community placements. This chapter encourages you to think about *how* best to learn and what it is that you need to know in order to practise. Authentic clinical placements, engaging with both practising clinical staff and patients, provide lots of informal learning opportunities alongside the formally acknowledged learning objectives in your course documentation. You will see examples of excellent care being provided, difficult patient interactions and team-work actually happening. You should take time to discuss these with your peers in confidential settings.

TASK

Consider a patient interaction that went exceptionally well and discuss with your peers why you think it was good.

Remember significant critical events can be of a positive nature as well as negative.

Medical students have been called 'test-wise' highlighting the importance of prioritising learning what you need to know to pass your examinations. Your progression along the course is important, and rightly so, but learning what you need to know to prepare to be the very best doctor can also be important, and community placements can play a vital role in this. Should you learn something because it will be examined, or because it is inherently interesting, or significantly relevant to patient care?

Many students, either at the start of their course or when they first enter the main clinical component of their studies, struggle getting the right balance between studying for their examinations and learning about clinical medicine. The amount of information and the lack of time do not seem compatible with learning what is required. Medical students therefore frequently become very strategic in how and what they decide to learn, often prioritising book learning rather than patient contact. Spending time in community placements will help you get the right balance between book learning and clinical practice. In general practice you will find opportunities to appreciate the context of the science you are learning, see the linkages between various disciplines and begin applying what you know to solve real-life clinical problems. Presenting clinical material so that the relevant knowledge you need to know is integrated into authentic real- life scenarios helps you appreciate what it is you do need to know to be a doctor, as well as pass your examinations.

To illustrate this we can think of a common presentation of a patient, Mr. Brown, a 61-year-old publican, who you see with your GP tutor during morning surgery. He has 2 weeks history of increasing shortness of breath and productive cough. His spirometry, done by the practice nurse last year, confirmed established chronic obstructive pulmonary disease (COPD). You notice from the computer screen that he has smoked since he was a teenager. Engaging with this patient presents multiple learning opportunities. Seeing Mr. Brown's spirometry results, and being able to interpret the findings, confirms your understanding of lung function, and highlights the link between the physiology you have been taught in lectures and practicals and its clinical relevance. You can easily practise taking a simple respiratory history, which is important in identifying the possible diagnosis before investigation, and in patients with an established diagnosis of COPD to monitor the progression of the disease, and effectiveness of any medication.

Depending on your experience you can take a full history and perform an appropriate clinical examination, present your findings and discuss a possible management plan with both the patient and your tutor. You will know that continued smoking has serious implications for Mr. Brown's prognosis and you need to explain this in an acceptable way to the patient.

Using evidence-based medical information and effective communication skills to improve patient outcomes is a challenge for students and their qualified practising medical tutors. To have an opportunity to

TASK

Consider how best to approach patients in discussing how they could modify their behaviour to improve their lifestyles and reduce risks to their health.

Ask your tutor to observe you discussing with a patient such behaviour modification advice, such as giving up smoking and receive some feedback.

Use the information from Chapter 2 (Cycle of Change) as you prepare for this work.

practice such activities facilitates your understanding of the synergistic relationship between theory and practice, and how best to learn what you need to know in order to both pass the examinations and be a good doctor. Authentic patient scenarios, such as the example above, provide opportunities to explore the multidisciplinary nature of investigation and treatment of conditions and provide opportunities for you to learn about the epidemiology and public health issues.

Your responsibilities at the end of your placement

A review meeting should be planned at the end of the placement. This isn't just the time to receive your assessment grades and complete any necessary paperwork, but it is also an opportunity to discuss what you have learnt, whether you have fulfilled your personal as well as formal learning objectives and how confident you feel about moving on.

Your tutors, like you, have an agenda, they have to complete an annual appraisal and will need to demonstrate they have achieved the goals they set with their appraiser, they will be looking for feedback from you as evidence that they have provided a good learning experience, they do not want to receive unconstructive critical feedback or complaints. In our experience tutors are particularly irked when students nod benignly or mumble 'it's all fine' or the equivalent when asked directly by tutors how the placement is going; only to later complain bitterly about their experience to the medical school either in person or via placement evaluation questionnaires. So, you have a professional responsibility to inform a practice through your tutor if things haven't gone so well and how the experience could be improved.

Ideally through regular contact with your tutor they should have had some prior notification and opportunity to put these things right before the end of the attachment but this isn't always possible. It's particularly important to outline whether you feel you have had sufficient opportunity, time and support in achieving your learning objectives. Conversely if your attachment has gone well then please do tell your tutor and the staff.

In the same way that tutors should complete a fair assessment of you, with an explanation of how they came to grade you as they did, at the end of your placement you should provide constructive feedback for your tutors. Schools will differ in how they collect placement evaluation from students but most will have an electronic questionnaire which may or may not be anonymous, it can be wearing to be asked to provide feedback on all teaching but do remember that in a few years time you will be asking your students to provide you with feedback so you can improve your teaching and so you have the all-important evidence for your appraisal.

A final word that it is your responsibility to relay any significant concerns you may have regarding the patient safety to your medical school. Your school will have a policy in place to deal with this and advise you.

Summary

In this chapter we have explored how to make the most from your community placements starting with the necessary preparations beforehand, tips for your learning while in placements and advice following your attachments. We have looked at your responsibilities as a professional to yourself, your colleagues and your patients – both in terms of personal safety, adequate planning and confidentiality. We have explored how best to prepare for the placement and what to expect from the placement, team and tutor. We have specifically helped you plan for the first meeting with your tutor, explained what a learning needs assessment is and how it can help. We have offered practical advice about how best to learn on clinical placements and will discuss this more in the following chapters. Finally we have offered advice to ensure that the placement is finished in a careful, considered and professional manner.

References

Ausubel D, Novak J and Hanesian H (1978) Educational Psychology: A Cognitive View. New York: Holt Rinehart & Winston, 163.

Cosgrove E (2006) The Challenge of Professionalism: Environment and Assessment. http://gec.kmu.edu.tw/gec2/conf/951209/file/06-Ellen_Cosgrove.pdf. Accessed 26 June 2014.

Eraut M (1994) Developing Professional Knowledge and Competence. London: The Falmer Press.

GMC (2009) Medical Students: Professional Values and Fitness to Practice. http://www.gmc-uk.org/education/undergraduate/professional_behaviour.asp. Accessed 31 March 2014.

GMC (2011) Clinical Placements for Medical Students – Advice Supplementary to Tomorrow's Doctors 2009. http://www.gmc-uk.org/static/documents/content/Clinical_placements_for_medical_students_1114.pdf. Accessed 28 March 2014.

GMC (2013) Duties of a Doctor. http://www.gmc-uk.org/guidance/good_medical_practice/duties_of_a_doctor.asp. Accessed 31 March 2014.

Luft J and Ingham H (1950) The Johari window, a graphic model of interpersonal awareness. Proceedings of the western training laboratory in group development. UCLA, Los Angeles.

Spencer J (2003) Teaching about professionalism. Medical Education 37: 288–289.

Chapter 4 **Active learning in the consultation**

With Catie Nagel

Introduction

In Chapter 1 we looked at the unique potential of learning medicine in primary care. You could learn all of medicine, and indeed all of life. This chapter will focus on learning how best to engage with patients, how to learn from them in a consultation, how to make the most of learning in this setting and how to be become an excellent communicator across a variety of challenging scenarios.

By the end of this chapter you should be able to:

- develop ideas on how to stay engaged and active in the consultation
- develop ideas of how to work with your tutor to stay involved and useful during your placement
- better understand the structure and content of consultations
- develop confidence to learn from and within more complex consultations.

The ability to communicate well with patients and colleagues is more than a desirable character trait. Good communication skills are an essential element of professional practice and therefore are vital to being a good doctor (General Medical Council, 2013). Consultation is the medium by which we not only come to a conclusion about the medical diagnosis and offer a management plan, but also develop an understanding of our patients and their lives. That is not to say that many secondary care physicians are not skilled consulters or that all GPs will be getting it right all of the time, but a considerable amount of

---

How to Succeed on Primary Care and Community Placements, First Edition.
David Pearson and Sandra Nicholson.
© 2016 John Wiley & Sons, Ltd. Published 2016 by John Wiley & Sons, Ltd.

research and educational time is dedicated to this aspect of medical practice within general practitioner training.

So, you have arrived at your surgery and met the practice manager and lead GP. What next? How can you make sure you enjoy and learn from the consultations you will sit in, and not be the student moaning to friends later that you had to sit in the corner and listen. That can be really boring, and make it really hard to learn anything. But you can change that!

> When I was a third-year medical student I remember clearly being presented with the terrifying task of taking my first primary care history. When faced with my rabbit-in-the-headlights facial expression, my tutor used the reassuring phrase: 'Don't worry, just act like you think a doctor should act'. Sound advice indeed. What followed was probably, to date, the worst consultation I have ever conducted. I giggled and grinned all the way through (my then usual response to stress). I hardly managed to gather one iota of useful information and certainly had no idea of how to proceed to a management plan. I still cringe when I think about it and wish I could somehow find that patient and apologise for my very un-doctor-like behaviour. However, I have carried that advice with me and whenever I'm faced with a new situation or I'm unsure what to do I go back to those wise words.
>
> (Catie)

Learning objectives, learning plans

Imagine, it's Monday morning, 9 a.m. (or maybe earlier!). You are sitting in the corner of a booked surgery. How will you learn from the 20 patients who will come through the door; presenting with multiple morbidity, complex problems, trivial problems, social problems, and all of whom the doctor already seems to know? Not easy and quite different from the hospital setting, where patients tend to present with defined problems, and well-rehearsed stories. But, real-life medicine nonetheless. Enjoy it.

First, you should already have a learning plan (see Chapter 3). Use it. Make sure your tutor knows what it is. Focus on what you really want to learn today, whether it is communication skills, how to manage asthma, how to examine eyes or something else. You can't learn everything, and you need to be able to make sense of complicated patients and consultations.

Second, listen and be prepared to learn, be prepared to be amazed. Patients will surprise you whether medically or socially or in terms of how they perceive or cope with illness. Have an open and receptive mind.

TASK: ENGAGING YOUR TUTOR – USING YOUR LEARNING PLAN

Suggest your tutor looks at your learning plan.
   Make sure he/she helps write it.
   Make sure he/she is aware of your prior learning, the stage of the course, the medical school's placement objectives, and if they are not sure, gently provide the information or direct them to the medical school website. This is really important.

Learning consultation skills

Are communication skills the same as consultation skills? Are we about to really confuse you? The short answer is – no, they are different, and we hope not!

In early years at medical school you will learn to communicate in a medical context. You will probably use Calgary Cambridge (Silverman *et al.*, 2004) – most schools do. You will know all about asking open questions, listening, summarising and maintaining empathy in the face of incredulity! That is all good, and can be learned with simulated patients and is best honed on real patients in the ward, clinics or here in surgery settings. Practise them, be an active learner, make mistakes along the way. What you might do in later clinical years though, especially in GP placements, is to really learn to consult. The consultation is a process which usually involves at least one 'expert' (Tuckett *et al.*, 1985) and has a purpose or an aim. The aim may not be clear from the start, but without one, you will be engaging in a discussion, a conversation or a chat! There may be several aims, sometimes referred to as 'agendas' within the consultation and these can come from a number of places – the patient, the doctor or a relative (Marvel *et al.*, 2013). A skilled consulter will be aware of these tensions and will work to navigate the best path, while keeping the patient at the heart of the process. It is no accident that the consultation is sometimes referred to as a 'journey' (Neighbour, 2005); try not to leave your patient behind or vice versa!

Understanding the consultation

You may already have learned a wealth of information about communicating with patients and about the components of a doctor–patient consultation. However, your time at the primary care placements is your chance to really embed this knowledge and start to become a good consulter yourself. This will be as important to you as a future surgeon as it would be in psychiatry, general practice or public health.

While revising your consultation skills, keep in mind the following (Neighbour, 2005; Silverman *et al.*, 2004)

- Remember *rapport building* (How the doctor introduces themselves to the patient and consultation, what effect does it have? Is it important and is it done differently in general practice?)
- Remember to ask *open questions* to gather broad information at the start and *closed questions* to check information, especially key facts (Please just tell me exactly where the pain was – point to the spot; am I right you said you had blood in the urine before the pain started?).
- Remember *check patient understanding* – whether the tutor is there or not (Just tell me what you thought caused the headache. Why do you think your child doesn't like school?)
- Practise *summarising* – whether to the patient ("Let me just check this – Abdul is 3 now, he has always been bad with his poos but in the last month he is only doing hard ones and sometimes there is blood.") or tutor ("OK, this is a 43-year-old lady who works in Tesco on the checkout, she came today to check her blood pressure because she has been having headaches and her mum died of a stroke at her age.").
- Practise *handing over* – ask your tutor to let you explain to the patient how to take tablets that are prescribed, or what the plan is if they don't work and the patient doesn't feel better.

There is a large quantity of information on communication and consultation skills. We highlight references particularly pertinent for community placements in the Reference Section (end of chapter).

The art of consultation

This is 'learning to drive' time. Being a good consulter involves starting to take the individual components of Calgary Cambridge or other consultation models for granted. It will come through practising and putting it all together. Rapport will be built instinctively; summarising will seem like second nature, handing over to the patient, part of what you do without thinking. Your primary care placements are the best setting to learn this. How do we help you there?

1 Learn the theory. GPs are good at this stuff. It is what they do. Neighbour's (2005, pp. 13–21) five 'checkpoints' in the consultation (Box 4.1) make a useful aide memoir to help you actively observe consultations. GPs build rapport, do the main consultation, hand over, safety net and (hopefully) look after themselves as they care for the patient.

2 Observe consultation skills in practice – take Neighbour's book with you and watch closely. None of the models of behaviour are perfect, but you'll see the component parts of Neighbour – and start to appreciate the skill of consulting.

3 Have a go, do it and practice, practice, practice. That's where placements in primary care really help – if you make them work for you. Be keen, say you want to practice, ask for feedback, think about the different bits of the consultation – and practice them in turn. GP tutors love keen students, and love keen, knowledgeable informed students even more.

Box 4.1 Neighbour's Five Checkpoints (Neighbour, 2005)

Checkpoint 1 – 'Connecting'
Checkpoint 2 – 'Summarising'
Checkpoint 3 – 'Handover'
Checkpoint 4 – 'Safety-netting'
Checkpoint 5 – 'Housekeeping'

Engaging with patients, introductions, information, consent

Engaging with patients

I hope it is self-evident from your medical school that you are expected to say 'hello' to patients, be polite. Introduce yourself as a medical student. This is as important in a GP surgery, whether with the nurse or patient or at reception, as it is in a hospital. Indeed in GP surgeries patients are a bit more their usual selves, a bit more empowered and might well pull you up for being rude if you don't introduce yourself (if not your tutor will).

But, that's all just good manners, or is it? Building rapport, which includes a good introduction, demonstrates mutual respect. Mutual respect builds trust and is arguably essential to allow an interchange of sensitive information (Bowling *et al.*, 2013; Martin *et al.*, 2013). Dr. Kate Granger's '#hellomynameis' campaign further highlights the importance of this initial introduction.

And more than just simple introductions, ask something about your patient as a person. After all 'Tomorrow's doctors' implores you to explore the physical, social and psychological aspects of disease for a good reason – they interlink and are often of equal importance.

> One of my most useful pieces of advice was from an excellent GP trainer and a font of wisdom. 'Always find something out about your patient', by which he meant the person in front of you, not the illness they may have presented with. That has served me in good stead. Finding out the patient with the Eastern European name fled Nazi Germany in 1938 because they were a Jew being persecuted offers a dramatic insight across all future encounters. You are more informed, the patient is impressed you are inquisitive and care about them. Finding out the tearful looking Mum has just lost her Dad is an important moment, even if she has come for more nappy cream for the baby. Not because you can ease her pain, just because you have engaged and listened. As a medical student you will often have more time with the patient to explore such things and offer insights for the GP or nurse.
>
> (David)

Introductions and information

It is worth checking with your tutor at the start of a surgery whether the GP will introduce you or whether you should introduce yourself when the patient arrives. If the GP has collected the patient from the waiting room it is sometimes hard to tell if they've remembered to tell the patient that they've got a student in and it can be quite hard to interrupt once they've started the consultation.

It is also worth exploring whether to be introduced as a medical student or a student doctor. You will be listened to more if the latter is used – but is it fair, or does it mislead patients? Your medical school might have a view, but perhaps a good rule is that in early clinical years, you are referred to as a 'medical student' and in later years, especially final year, as a 'student doctor'.

What about consent for your being in the room?

It is important. It is good practice (GMC, 2011). It is too rarely asked for. Your host practice will have a system of informing patients that it teaches medical students, including printed information at the reception desk and in the practice leaflet informing patients specifically about your presence in the surgery. The practice should let patients know 'A student is present with Dr. J this morning, is that OK with you?' The GP should then ask again when they call the patient in. This doesn't always happen, and patients don't like that (which affects how they respond to future students). Sometimes, perhaps practices bend too far to be patient centred – after all within the NHS, some might argue that it is the duty of the patients to be involved with teaching, to give something back. Some arrangement that is neutral would be nice – but you can do your bit. If a patient is clearly uncomfortable, just ask if they mind you being there. They'll appreciate that, as will your tutor who might be so embroiled listening to the story that he/she may have forgotten to ask.

Working with patients

Patients are increasingly 'co-producers of health' (Wensing and Elwyn, 2003). Gone are the days where patients were told what to do, and expect that they would listen to everything. It is your responsibility as a future clinician to facilitate this process. Current assessment at undergraduate and postgraduate level will, to varying degrees, assess the candidate's ability to practise patient-centred medicine (RCGP, 2011). To practise patient-centred medicine you must first understand what is meant by this:

Examples of patient-centred behaviour	Examples of doctor-centred behaviour
Seeks to understand what beliefs the patient has about the condition	Tells the patient what condition they have
Seeks to understand what the patient thinks has contributed to the condition	Tells the patient what they have or haven't done to contribute to the condition
Seeks to understand what the patient believes your role is	Undertakes the role felt most appropriate for that patient
Considers how the patient's environment or lifestyle may have contributed to the condition	Has a blanket approach to diagnosis regardless of what environment the patient lives in or comes from
Considers the condition in the context of the patient's life – what are the short- and long-term impacts?	Expects the patient to comply with advice or treatment regardless of beliefs, social and environmental pressures
Seeks to understand and considers the patient's preferences for information and shared decisionmaking	Involves or does not involve the patient in the decision-making process regardless of preference
Doctor and patient develop common therapeutic goals	Doctor tells the patient what to do

The word 'condition' is used as patients may come with a variety of requests and/or problems. There may not always be a biomedical disease to consider or a mental health problem, therefore this word is intended to encompass the paradigms of disease, illness, life events, problems and concerns. There is a wealth of information on patient-centredness. The preceding table is inspired by previous work, and some consultation models that you might be aware of: Byrne and Long (1976); Helman (1981); Pendelton *et al.* (1984); Mead and Bower (2000) and the BARD model (Warren, 2002) which discusses the role of the doctor during the consultation.

A model describes how something is done. Post-qualification none of us consult strictly to one particular model – these are frameworks with elements that can be drawn on from time to time. You may, however, be asked to demonstrate the entirety of one particular model (most commonly a modified version of Calgary-Cambridge) during assessment.

Seeking to understand the patient's 'I.C.E' (Ideas, Concerns and Expectations) has become a familiar utterance in undergraduate consultation skills sessions. This is particularly vital when on community placements due to the undifferentiated nature of presentations in primary care (especially to GPs) and the importance of understanding the patient's agenda because they have chosen to come to us rather than being referred into a service. Ask yourself if you are truly doing this or merely paying lip-service to the acronym? Phrases such as 'What do you think might be going on?' or 'What did you expect me to do today?' can be helpful when you're starting out, but if used without thought, these can have negative consequences and result in lack of engagement from the patient and a rejection of the whole process. If the patient replies 'I don't know, you're the doctor!' ask yourself why this might be. Could you have rephrased your question or is this patient ill-prepared for taking on a shared responsibility? Patients don't always come with a pre-formed idea of what they think is wrong and what they want you to do. They may not want to be involved in the decision-making process. This is fine. We certainly wouldn't advocate pushing for patient involvement if they are not ready for it, but you may want to consider why this might be.

Flexibility is extremely important if you want to become a skilled consulter. There is no 'one-size-fits-all' approach. At times it may in fact be appropriate to behave in a doctor-centred manner and each consultation is likely to require elements of both approaches. To give you an example; our patients may request something of us that we are unable to give either because of lack of resources or because it is not felt to be in the patient's best interest (GMC, 2013, Good Medical Practice/Duties of a Doctor). In these situations we should try our best to find an outcome that meets both the doctor's and the patient's agendas, but we might have to resort, in the end, to a very doctor-centred 'No'.

TASK

Think about a time when you have been to the GP or have been with a friend or a family member.

Was it a good or a bad experience? What made this so?

How does it relate to the current practice?

How involved were you (or the friend/family member) in the consultation and decision-making process?

Active learning in the consultation

TASK: PREPARING TO GET INVOLVED

You should be actively involved in the consultations. If you aren't you could suggest to your tutor that the surgery is set up to allow observed consultations (see below), and for experienced students see if there is an extra room to facilitate your involvement with supervised autonomous consultations (see below).

In the United Kingdom GPs are paid to provide time for teaching. You may still need to be a little assertive to keep your placement experiences active and rewarding when many pressures compete with your tutor's time. Be respectful of those time pressures though.

Active listening

A lot of the time in your primary care placement you'll be in with the GP or nurse tutor observing their consultations. It is vital to make this an active, involved process. Let's see how you can help facilitate this (and what to do if it isn't).

Not all GPs are good listeners all the time; time pressure, anxiety and outside influences can affect communication, but most GPs gain their information from listening carefully. As students you can also learn a lot by watching, by active listening and by observing exactly what range of information and techniques your tutor(s) use to elicit information.

In early placements it is common practice to observe other doctors consulting. If you are not careful this can very quickly become a passive process whereby you end up sitting and daydreaming without taking in any useful learning experiences. Role modelling has already been mentioned (Chapter 3) as a valuable tool in the development of consultation skills and professional attitudes – so now is the time to sit up and take note. You may decide that the person you are watching is not someone you would like to model yourself on, however you can learn just as much by watching behaviours that you do NOT wish to emulate (and reflecting on why that might be the case).

Active observation

David Hockney, arguably Britain's greatest living artist, when writing about his art, makes a clear distinction between the act of looking at something and active observation. As an artist he has to *really* look and understand what he sees to be able to interpret the scene and reproduce it. This is applicable to clinical practice, as research has shown that by training students in observation skills using fine art, they are better able to recognise clinical patterns and identify X-ray anomalies (Dolev *et al.*, 2001; Shapiro *et al.*, 2006). You must not only learn to look, but to see. Early observed consultations will be a blur of apparent short cuts and random exchanges. You need techniques to break down what you see and help you actively observe and understand the encounters which unfold.

Focus on one person

Now that you know what you are looking for, you will be able to make the most of your observed surgeries. It is a good idea to focus on one person at a time when you start watching others consult. For each consultation choose who you are going to focus on prior to the start and make a concerted effort to vary your focus with each new consultation. The following table can be used as a guide to what combinations you could use to structure your observation, for example, a relative's body language throughout a consultation – did it vary and what was this in response to?

Active observation in the consultation

Who to watch?	What to watch for?	When watching the doctor/nurse
Doctor/nurse	Body language	Clinician-centred behaviour
Patient	Words and phrases used	Patient-centred behaviour
Relative/carer	Who is in control of the consultation? Speed, volume and tone of voice (s)	Use of the computer and other aids

Make notes and be specific
If the doctor leaned forward in his/her chair, what happened immediately before this? Write down or remember what happened prior
to this action and think about it at the end. If the patient came
across as anxious, what precisely did you see or hear that made you
come to this decision? When observing words and phrases try to
make a note of exactly what these words were, not the meaning you
deduce from them. It is important to go through this process so that
you can learn how misunderstandings arise and how you can prevent them. Think about the meanings of these words and phrases at
the end of the consultation – could they have been interpreted in a
different way?

Active involvement in consultation
Where you sit is really important
Ideally the GP tutor will insist you sit within a triangle, so you are
involved and have a good view of both the patient and the tutor. Be
active in this – pull in your chair and have a presence. Most tutors will
want you to show initiative and interest. Sometimes this isn't possible:
there may be too few chairs, relatives and carers, children or interrup-
tions through examinations. But stay involved and in the centre of the
action – get up, be active, ask questions, have a presence; involvement
drives learning.

Example 1: Nicely out of the way, but too far from the action for any meaningful involvement. May come across as disinterested. Hard to stay engaged.

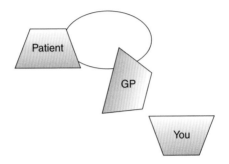

Example 2: Close to the action, but watch your spacing. Personal space is important. Unless a close personal acquaintance, most people need one metre space between them and the person they are speaking to. Too close and you will make the person feel uncomfortable and even threatened. This is particularly important if someone is suffering with some mental health problems.

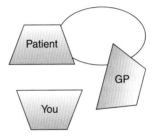

Example 3: Better, but the patient may feel threatened, as if you and the GP are 'ganging up' against them.

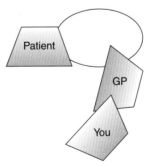

Example 4: Probably our preference for this room lay out. Close enough that the GP tutor can involve you, but not so close to the patient that you may make them feel inhibited or threatened.

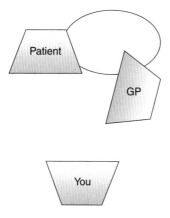

Ask questions

It is dull for tutors to have a quiet student. Good tutors will engage with you, but we all have bad days so you can help. Be prepared; think ahead of the surgery about what you need to learn, today, this week, this module. Ask questions! General practice is so general that you can find a relevant thing in every surgery, probably in every patient. A clear relevant question about every patient will add up to a wealth of learning, so much better than looking up the Internet or reading books. Try it. 'Why is that lady on a beta blocker not an ACE inhibitor?' 'How long will you continue the

---

TASK: GETTING ACTIVELY INVOLVED

A good student will show initiative. A good tutor will have time set aside for you, actively observe you, encourage you to see patients on your own, have a spare room available – and give you a focussed task. 'Talk with Mrs. Jones while I see the next patient, but I want you to find out exactly how this condition affects her day-to-day life'. If you are lucky, appreciate the skills of your tutor and thank him/her. If you aren't properly engaged, maybe ask subtly 'some of my friends are seeing more patient by themselves, could I have that chance?' 'What exactly do you want me to concentrate on?'

fluoxetine for?' 'What do you think about cognitive behavioural therapy (CBT) in depression?' A good tutor will bounce questions back, but you will be engaged and learning, and become a better doctor as a result.

Student-led consultations

The previous section looked at how even observed consultations can be rewarding learning experiences. However, what will really help you learn is getting more involved with the running of some or all consultations. This is less feasible in early years at medical school, but should become an increasing feature of later clinical placements. With prior planning patients should expect this to happen and will often enjoy it as much as you will.

Student-focussed consultations

Observing a good doctor or nurse is valuable, but ideally your tutor will (or should, especially if he/she borrows this volume) keep stopping his/her consultation to pass the baton to you – 'OK Mrs. XX, now I will ask Jane to just listen to your chest and tell me what she finds', 'OK Mr. YY, I now have a good idea of what is going on, but let's just let Jane summarise what we have found'. The key point is that a good tutor should keep focussing on you and your learning needs, but do so respectfully and with the patient's consent. You can help by asking 'Do you mind if I try to summarise?', 'Do you mind if I check the urine' and so on.

Student-led consultations

Even better than student-focussed consultations is getting the chance to run a part of or all consultations. If your tutor doesn't suggest it, just ask. Take his/her seat. Start the consultation (with permission from the patient, and tutor, of course!). Or, with arrangement, swap half way: 'OK, now we've taken a history and examined you, I'll just let Kamal have my seat, summarise what we have found and say what we do next…'. That will keep you listening, focussed and involved. Through a balanced use of student-led consultations, you'll be able to practice history taking, examination, summarising, giving information, sharing decision making and other vital skills of being a doctor.

Problems, pitfalls and suggested solutions

How to consult when you don't know anything

When you start consulting independently you may find that it all feels like a real muddle as you are trying to assimilate what the patient is telling you with your current level of medical knowledge. Don't be fooled into thinking that you can only improve your consultation skills once you have learned more of the medical facts. The truth is that as medical science is a rapidly advancing field we all find ourselves in situations where we have a deficit of knowledge from time to time (either because the research in this area is inconclusive or due to a personal blind spot) – it is therefore important to know how to progress in a consultation even if you don't have a firm diagnosis. The Royal College of General Practitioners calls this 'tolerating uncertainty' (RCGP, 2010b). Although this could be viewed as a postgraduate skill, it is important to dispel the myth that once you qualify you will know everything!

Maintaining structure can be more of a challenge. You may be familiar with several models which will help you with this. The 'hospital' biomedical history-taking model (presenting complaint, history of presenting complaint, past medical history, family history, drug history, allergy history, social history and systemic enquiry) and the Calgary-Cambridge model are the two models taught most commonly in medical school. We recommend the book *Skills for Communicating with Patients* by Silverman *et al.* (2004) for more information – but there are many others available (see Reference Section at the end of the chapter).

An analogy we find useful is Roger Neighbour's 'Two Heads' (Neighbour, 2005). Neighbour describes the 'Organiser' – the part of your brain that uses logical processes, analyses information and sets goals, and the 'Responder' which is intuitive and focussed on feelings and emotions. For a successful consultation both heads need to be operational, you must develop the ability to flit between the two. The 'Organiser' is responsible for structure and timing as well as calling upon medical knowledge and has a lot to do, especially when you have trouble recalling biomedical facts!

Fears, concerns and emotions

Techniques that can help with responding to concerns are to do with authenticity. Some might argue that you can't teach empathy, but what we can learn is how to display or communicate it. If you take an interest in what the patient is saying and try to understand the situation from their point of view, then you are already more than half way there. Things that might prevent you from responding to a concern appropriately include embarrassment or a fear that you won't find the right words, but actually, what makes us as tutors (and examiners) cringe more than anything is false reassurance. What we mean by this is reassurance that sounds as if it is not meant or is actually inappropriate. For example:

> Mrs. Davies has been suffering with pain on defecation associated with a small amount of bright red rectal bleeding each time she passes a motion. She is in her early 30s and has just had her second baby. She has suffered from piles previously. She appears anxious and you manage to elicit the fact that she is worried about cancer. You say 'Oh, don't worry about that Mrs. Davies! You most likely have piles, it is very rare for a person as young as you to get bowel cancer'. Of course, she will be relieved to hear this. This may be the case, she most likely does have piles, BUT can you justify this response yet? You have not examined her, she may have a strong history of hereditary bowel cancer, she may even be concealing additional information from you such as weight loss as she fears it is the 'Big C' and is in a state of denial and avoidance. People don't always act in the way you might expect.

Remember the mnemonic 'ALL EARS' (Harrison *et al.*, 2007)

A – Acknowledge concern	Show the patient that you have heard his/her concern by repeating or summarising
L – Legitimise concern	Show the patient that you accept his/her concern. Do not dismiss it as silly even if it seems implausible
L – Listen	Encourage the patient to expand on the reasons for the concern
E – Empathise	Show the patient that you are trying to see things from his/her perspective
A – Avoid (premature or false) R – Reassurance	Avoid giving reassurance before you have obtained and assessed all the information needed and are sure you have the knowledge to do so
S – Summarise	Check that you have understood the patient correctly, so you can then move on

And finally, how not to learn in a consultation

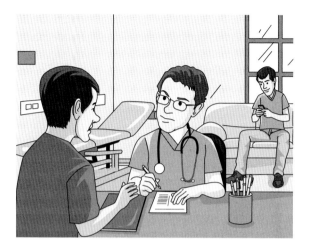

What won't help you to learn is to be in a corner, passive, unengaged, avoiding eye contact, on your mobile or even reading a book (although the occasional glance at the relevant Oxford Handbook or BNF might be acceptable!). Get involved, stay involved, engage!

Complex consultations for the later clinical years

Not all consultations involve a single articulate patient coming in with a simple medical problem. That would be nice for learning and for the doctor. It rarely happens. A whole range of complexities frequently get in the way. This section covers some of those, how to deal with them, how to learn from them and when to quietly retire and observe from the corner.

Consultations with children

Consultations with children make up between 20% and 25% of workload (Saxena *et al.*, 1999; RCGP, 2010a) and the rate is hugely variable depending on practice demographics. Many GPs love this work – some consider these as 'quick consultations', but we (the authors) have always thought they are often longer and more complex.

Consider this. How much does the child understand? How much should the child be involved or empowered? Who is the most needy patient; the mother or her child? New mothers may be depressed, isolated or anxious, and this may present with frequent attendances for the children. How do you allay anxiety if you are also anxious? How do you cope with three unruly children and adequately examine the one who is unwell?

For learning, the previous principles apply. What do you want to learn? What do you need to learn? Engage with your tutor to learn it. That might again be examination skills or about common childhood problems. It might be learning about common parental anxieties – the small child, persistent cradle cap, itches and allergies, knock knees and flat feet. It might not be brain surgery or ER – but this is why families visit doctors and this is what they worry about.

If nothing else use your time in general practice to make sure you are really confident about communicating with and examining children. See lots of children, draw pictures, make paper airplanes, smile, play and enjoy it. Learn from experienced GPs and nurses. You will suddenly appreciate these skills in your objective structured clinical examination (OSCE) and finals, as well as later life.

Consultations across language barriers

Half a million people come to the United Kingdom every year to stay long term. Many will not have English as a first language. Some may speak very minimal English or sometimes none at all. As future doctors you will need to learn how to best communicate when language creates a challenge. When a significant language barrier is in place, both clinicians and patients find the consultation more satisfying if an interpreter is used, rather than trying to make do with simple English (Li *et al.*, 2010). If a professional interpreter is used there will be a lesser likelihood of misdiagnosis and an increased chance that the patient will understand the advice given or know how to take their medication. Use of a professional face-to-face interpreter in these situations should be regarded as the gold standard. We hope you will have the chance to practice consultations both with patients who have limited English and use trained interpreters. 'Triadic' consultations (that use interpreters) are an advanced skill and even qualified doctors find these tricky.

If you are in later clinical years and have an opportunity to talk with patients with limited English when no interpreter is present, you might consider the following:

- Speak slowly and clearly, use short sentences
- Ask one question at a time (and wait for the response)
- Avoid use of the past tense as much as possible, for example, can you, were you, did you?
- Gesture, point and draw diagrams to aid understanding
- Examine the patient more readily as the history will be of variable quality
- Use eye contact and non-verbal gestures to convey active listening, but be aware when this might not be culturally appropriate (in some cultures direct eye contact is felt to be disrespectful, e.g., Aboriginal culture)
- Where 'ad-hoc' interpreters are used (family members or friends) be aware of issues around confidentiality
- Speak to the patient directly, rather than the interpreter (e.g., 'where is the pain?' rather than 'ask her where the pain is?')
- If using a telephone interpreter, aim to use a hands-free mode (e.g., monitor or speakerphone) to avoid passing the receiver back and forth
- Be attentive for non-verbal cues. Reflect these back (e.g., you look worried, is there anything else you want to talk about?)

Confidentiality in the consultation

Remember throughout your placement you must respect patient's confidentiality and disclose information only on a 'need to know basis'. This is reinforced elsewhere in this book, but within the consultation ensure you do not inadvertently reveal to a carer or relative something of a patient's past life – be extremely careful with information you receive or records you see (does your patient want their new boyfriend to know about past infections or terminations?).

Conflict

One thing which challenges us all as practicing clinicians is conflict. Conflict with us (patients are often upset is they don't get the treatment or the sick note they wanted), conflict between children and parents (the fine line between strictness and abuse is often touched upon in the consultation room), conflict between patient and carer (especially with

TASK: WHAT TO DO IF YOU ARE BORED

It may be despite your best efforts you are still sitting in the corner and passive. It may be the service demands, meaning your tutor simply hasn't had the chance to plan your teaching or encourage your active involvement on this particular occasion. If this happens, do three things:

1 Challenge yourself – what can I do to engage directly with patients, what can I offer to do to make learning more active or make myself part of the team?

2 Talk to the tutor or practice manager and raise your concerns directly (no one likes to hear concerns second hand).

3 If necessary raise your concerns early with your medical school/head of PC teaching or equivalent – it's no good raising concerns at the end of the placement when the medical school cannot do anything for you.

mental illness, often an outpouring of frustration or powerlessness such as with dementia). If you are upset or scared by what you see, talk with your tutor or peers. Learn from your experiences, but don't get stressed by them.

Summary

Your primary care placement is an ideal time to develop your consultation skills. You will have lots of opportunities to access patients under the close supervision from your clinical tutor, which oftentimes is one-to-one. Make the most of these opportunities and practice the skills you learn as much as possible on real patients, look for honest feedback and if things didn't go so well, take the time to reflect on what went wrong. The satisfaction that comes with development of these skills will not only benefit your future patients, but will also enhance your enjoyment of practicing medicine. There are a finite number of diagnoses that can be made, but an infinite number of variations as to how these conditions will present and affect those afflicted. Interest yourself in the lives of your patients and your job as a practitioner will always be varied and challenging.

References

Bowling, A., Rowe, G. and McKee, M. 2013. Patients' experiences of their healthcare in relation to their expectations and satisfaction: a population survey. Journal of the Royal Society of Medicine, 106 (4), 143–9.

Byrne, P.S. and Long, B.E.L. 1976. Doctors Talking to Patients. London: HMSO.

Dolev, J., Friedlaender, L. and Braverman, I. 2001. Use of fine art to enhance visual diagnostic skills. JAMA, 286, 1020.

General Medical Council. 2011. Clinical placement for medical students; advice supplementary to Tomorrow's Doctors (2009). [Online]. Available from: http://www.gmc-uk.org/static/documents/content/Clinical_placements_for_medical_students_1114.pdf. Accessed 8 April 2014.

General Medical Council. 2013. Good Medical Practice. Available from: http://www.gmc-uk.org/guidance/good_medical_practice.asp. Accessed 28 January 2015.

Harrison, C.J. and Wass, H.V. 2007. Learning to communicate using the framework. The Clinical Teacher, 4(3), 159–64.

Helman, C.G. 1981. Disease versus illness in general practice. Journal of Royal College of General Practitioners, 31, 548–52.

Li, S., Pearson, D. and Escott, S. 2010. Language barriers within primary care consultations: an increasing challenge needing new solutions. Education for Primary Care, 21(6), 385–91. Available at: http://www.ncbi.nlm.nih.gov/pubmed/21144177. Accessed 4 July 2015.

Martin, K.D., Roter, D.L., Beach, M.C., Carson, K.A. and Cooper, L.A. 2013. Physician communication behaviours and trust among black and white patients with hypertension. Medical Care, 51 (2), 151–7.

Marvel, K., Epstein, R.M., Flowers, K. and Beckman, H.B. 2013. Soliciting the patient's agenda have we improved? JAMA, 281 (3), 283–7.

Mead, N. and Bower, P. 2000. Patient-centeredness: a conceptual framework and review of the empirical literature. Social Science & Medicine, 51(7), 1087–110. Available at: http://www.ncbi.nlm.nih.gov/pubmed/11005395. Accessed 4 July 2015.

Neighbour, R. 2005. The Inner Consultation: How to Develop an Effective and Intuitive Consulting Style. Abingdon: Radcliffe.

Pendelton, D., Schofield, T., Tate, P. and Havelock, P. (1984) The Consultation: An Approach to Learning and Teaching. Oxford: OUP.

Royal College of General Practitioners. 2010a. Care of Children and Young People [Online]. Available from: http://www.rcgp.org.uk/~/media/Files/GP-training-and-exams/Curriculum-2012/RCGP-Curriculum-3-04-Children-and-Young-People.ashx. Accessed 8 April 2014.

Royal College of General Practitioners. 2010b. The Competence Framework: 6. Managing Medical Complexity and Promoting Health. http://www. rcgp-curriculum.org.uk/mrcgp/wpba/competence_framework.aspx. Accessed 4 July 2015.

Royal College of General Practitioners. 2011. Curriculum Statement 2: The General Practice Consultation [online]. Available from: http://www.rcgp-curriculum.org.uk/curriculum_documents/gp_curriculum_statements. aspx. Accessed 18 June 2012.

Saxena, S., Majeed, A. and Jones, M. 1999. Socioeconomic differences in childhood consultation rates in general practice in England and Wales: prospective cohort study. BMJ, 318, 642–6.

Shapiro, J., Rucker, L. and Beck, J. 2006. Training the clinical eye and mind: using the arts to develop medical students' observational and pattern recognition skills. Medical Education, 40, 263–8.

Silverman, J., Kurtz, S. and Draper, J. 2004. Skills for Communicating with Patients, 2nd Edition. Oxford: Radcliffe Medical Press.

Tuckett, D., Boulton, M., Olson, C. and Williams, A. 1985. Meetings Between Experts: An Approach to Sharing Ideas in Medical Consultations. London: Tavistock Publications.

Warren, E. 2006. An Introduction to BARD: A New Consultation Model. Outlined at: SkillsCascade.com.

Wensing, M. and Elwyn, G. 2003. Methods for incorporating patients' views in health care. BMJ, 326(7394), 877–879.

Chapter 5 **What to learn from the primary healthcare team**

With Will Spiring and Ann O'Brien

This chapter will look at the importance of the primary healthcare team (PHCT) and how to get the most out of working with it.

By the end of this chapter you should be able to:

- know who does what in the PHCT
- understand what you can learn from the team about medicine, patient care and teamwork
- understand how you can best learn clinical and procedural skills from the PHCT
- understand how you can use and encourage insight from across the team and from patients to strengthen your own professional development as a future doctor

It is our firm belief that time spent with a wide range of professionals making up the PHCTs is time well spent. Not only is it essential for you to understand how teams work and about the roles of a range of colleagues, but this is also a fantastic chance to learn knowledge and skills.

- *Knowledge* because nurses, physiotherapists, pharmacists and others hold a huge amount of specialist knowledge
- *Skills* because here is the place to develop or consolidate clinical skills and procedural skills essential to allow you to prepare for practice
- On top of this you'll become a better teamworker, better communicator and gain a variety of new perspectives on patient care.

We should at the outset highlight that we are talking here about two often distinct PHCTs. The first team you will work with is the one that

How to Succeed on Primary Care and Community Placements, First Edition.
David Pearson and Sandra Nicholson.
© 2016 John Wiley & Sons, Ltd. Published 2016 by John Wiley & Sons, Ltd.

is based in the practice or health centre, a small and often tight team of clinicians and support staff. The second team is the community-based PHCT who are often less closely aligned to the doctors who will tutor you, being more focussed on care for those who are housebound, with limited mobility or with specialist needs and looked after outside of surgeries (ranging from pregnancy to drug and alcohol problems to some mental health provision). Both teams offer rich learning opportunities and it is important to know and understand both the teams. Chapter 5 will focus mainly on learning within the practice-based PHCT, while Chapter 6 will focus on opportunities in wider community settings.

Introduction

The multidisciplinary team (MDT) that makes up the PHCT has always been at the heart of good community care and general practice. Consequently, for 'Tomorrow's Doctors' an understanding of what the PHCT is and how it works is an essential prerequisite for learning. In the United Kingdom this is an explicit curriculum requirement, that is, to develop teamwork skills and the need to understand the professional roles of team members (GMC, 2009a, Tomorrows Doctors Para 22). Placements early in medical school often focus on the team approach to care in the community.

Later on in the clinical years as a medical student, you need to be able to navigate the multidisciplinary landscape so you can take full advantage of what it has to offer in terms of education. The team

---

PCHT members

- Understand what knowledge and skills are needed to deliver areas of patient care they are working with on a daily basis
- Offer valuable perspectives on delivering holistic care in community settings.
- Reflection, supervision and mentorship is an integral part of their training and development
- Have a valuable insight into what can go wrong with patient care (learning from errors is a vital part of healthcare quality improvement).

can be a rich source of patient contact and related learning. For the medical student who can 'fit in' it provides many opportunities to practice clinical skills and test clinical knowledge from throughout the curriculum.

Being comfortable with how the team works, understanding what each member does and discussing with your tutor what you can realistically expect to learn from your placement will help prepare you to both learn and work in this busy environment. There is no substitute for fully involving yourself within the team. Spending quality time on these placements will prepare you to work and develop professionally throughout your future career.

Professional behaviour in a team

Working within the team becomes a required skill in its own right in preparation for professional practice. It is common to have course outcomes related to the team itself. Some examples of these are given in the table from different UK medical schools.

Year 1	Discuss the role of the PHCT in support and treatment of patients whose social circumstances impact their health	Barts and The London
Year 3	Gain some understanding of the skill mix and interprofessional working in general practice	Bristol
Year 4	Describe the members and roles of the PHCT and the important principles of teamwork	Queens Belfast
Year 5	Establish rational and cost effective management plans, including therapeutics and prescribing, taking into consideration the role of the whole PHCT	Kings

While your own medical school will provide you with your own specific learning outcomes, knowledge of individual professional roles and how the team functions and works with patients are common themes. An understanding of teams working in terms of good communication and the professional behaviours that promote it are also important at undergraduate level. 'Tomorrow's Doctors' are universally assessed for an attitude that demonstrates the professional qualities that will enhance patient care through team working.

> Communicate clearly, sensitively and effectively with … colleagues from the medical and other professions, by listening, sharing and responding.
>
> GMC (2009a) Tomorrow's Doctors Para 15(a)

> Participate in a collaborative team-based model and with consulting health professionals in the care of patients; Work with others to assess, plan, provide and integrate care for individual patients or groups of patients.
>
> CFPC (2009) CANMEDS

Your primary care placement offers an ideal place to involve yourself in the PHCT (both practice and community based) and get to understand how it works. You will observe excellent teams in secondary care as well – renal care, cancer care, palliative care, anaesthesia and the emergency department spring to mind. Sometimes your placements in primary care may be longer and you may have more time with the various professionals involved. Use it wisely.

What is required of the professional is often defined in terms of knowledge, skills and attitude.

Knowledge of team working

You must know about the PHCT; in particular the roles of each member, what they do, what they don't do, how they were trained, how they keep up to date, how they relate to other team members.

You also need to know about how teams function in general. An effective team needs leadership, focus, an appropriate level of challenge and management of resources. Outside the specialist roles professionals play, with expertise from different disciplines, there are contributions individuals make to general team working. As a doctor within a clinical team, you will need to appreciate and contribute to meeting these requirements.

To operate professionally within a team you also need to know something about what can go wrong. Identifying risk will help you make your team practice safer.

Skills for team working

Skills required to work in a team are often seen as well aligned with those needed to be a good doctor. Communication, synthesizing information, providing feedback, problem solving and managing time and other resources effectively are all important. Of these, communication often provides a major challenge and poor quality of communication can quickly become a source of risk to patient safety. Within the PHCT, time must be taken to communicate the clinical information to the necessary team members in a timely manner. Availability of team members to each other for effective two-way communication is important. You will need to learn how to summarise relevant information, present it in an understandable form verbally and in writing and make decisions about the ethics and legal aspects of record keeping and confidentiality. The advantages and challenges of clinical information systems are explored in Chapter 7.

Attitudes to teamwork

Attitudes to teamwork impact your professionalism. Teams require open and two-way exchange of expertise with a willingness to learn from other professionals, patients and carers. There must be sharing of the team's successes and failures. It is clear that the general public and government have high expectations of medical professionals and demand a culture of openness when things go wrong (see *Learning from Mistakes*). An appreciation of, and alertness to, team members' contributions and needs is vital; as is an appreciation of operating in the

---

TASK: PARTICIPATING IN MULTIDISCIPLINARY TEAM MEETINGS

Make sure you attend or participate in multidisciplinary team meetings when you are on your primary care placement. Ask your tutor if this isn't timetabled.
- Who is involved in the team, and who is not?
- How patient focussed is the team and the discussion?
- Actively observe the range of contributions in the meet and listen to different perspectives.
- What are the points of agreement? What are the points of tension?

context of different members workload and pressures. The old adage there is no 'i' in team is true enough, but there must be plenty of 'eyes' and they all need to be open.

What the PHCT does

It will help if you have a basic understanding of each professional's role within the team. Starting with knowledge of the role each member plays, you can use the strengths of each member and their commitment to the team to help you learn. We have previously made a distinction between two main PHCTs you will encounter, the 'practice or health centre-based team' and the 'community healthcare team'. At best the two overlap and form one team; this varies from country to country.

Practice-based PHCTs: You will often be linked to a GP or family doctor on your placement, and in the United Kingdom and many other countries, you will be taught within the practice. The practice team will typically and vitally include practice nurses, nurse practitioners, pharmacists, healthcare assistants and sometimes physiotherapists and councillors. Not every practice will have each of these professionals, and many of these staff may be co-located outside GP surgeries.

The community PHCT operates in a wider context with patients supported by a variety of staff based out with practices, for example, community nurses including community matrons, district nurses, midwives, health visitors, Macmillan nurses, specialist nurses (e.g., diabetes, dementia and Parkinson's), community pharmacists, physiotherapists, occupational therapists, social workers and others you may have been more familiar with in hospital settings.

Increasingly the traditional boundaries between team members' roles are blurred. The best way to find out what people do is to ask them. There is often more heterogeneity within the community team than in the hospital setting, but your tutor should help ensure that your placement fulfils your learning outcomes; because placements are not identical it does not mean they are not equivalent.

Some key practice and community healthcare team roles are listed in the table.

Role	Training/career path (UK)	Educational involvement
Practice nurse		
Management of long-term conditions	3+ years for nurse registration (now degree level)	Many nurses will have educational mentoring qualification required for supervising nursing students
Health promotion advice	Further training for specific skills organised by employers, e.g.	Educational theory and theory of reflective practice has a prominent role in nurse training
Immunisation (children, adults and travellers)	1 year for specialist consultation skills such as minor illness or diabetes /respiratory/CVD	
Primary and secondary screening (e.g., cervical, STDs, diabetes, dementia)	1 year for independent prescribing status	
Contraception and sexual health		
Often involved in the clinical aspects of performance monitoring and quality improvement		
District nurse (community)		
Role being similar to practice nurse, but for housebound patients. Increasingly work delivered through clinics in health centres (e.g., dressings for those who are mobile). Often co-ordinating care in teams with District Nurse assistants (HCA's) and care agencies. May play a central role in palliative and terminal care	Nurse training plus specialist practitioner training (at least 1 year)	

(Continued)

(Continued)

Role	Training/career path (UK)	Educational involvement
Community specialist nurse Respiratory specialists; diabetes specialists; Parkinson's nurses; Wound management and tissue viability; substance misuse; renal and dialysis		
Community psychiatric nurse The community mental health team is a whole multidisciplinary team in itself. Community psychiatric nurses are often involved closely with the PHCT in the management of more stable long-term mental health difficulties		
Community midwife (UK) Responsible for care of uncomplicated pregnancies throughout the antenatal period, through birth to 28 days postnatally. May carry out postnatal infant checks. May manage the delivery either on the labour ward or at home	Basic qualified nurse training plus 18 months additional training Or 3 years direct entry training Further qualifications for carrying out extended roles such as new birth checks	Similar to nursing
Health visitor (UK) Most are specifically employed in the care of children and families under 5 years. Independent professionals who will monitor, promote the well-being of young families. Key role in safeguarding vulnerable children, and overseeing 'at risk registers'	Usually a nurse or midwifery background and then a further 1-year training	Most will have some formal mentoring qualification. Many have advanced educational qualifications, e.g., Masters level

Healthcare assistant (practice based) Carry out a number of health-related procedures usually with a defined work plan or protocol such as template or proforma data gathering, ECG or other technical procedures or phlebotomy	Varies. Most train on the job to gain QCT level 2/3.	Formal educational qualifications are unusual but many may be training to go onto other allied health professions
Social worker The role of social workers is as varied as that of the nurse or doctor. Those who work closely with the PHCT are usually specialised in vulnerable children or adults, mental health or elderly care. They usually form part of a targeted team such as rehabilitation or admissions prevention	Social work degree and professional qualification at honours (3 years) or masters level (2 years with relevant previous graduate degree and experience)	
Practice manager (UK) Responsibility for practice systems, staffing, HR, financial matters, governance, complaints and statutory responsibilities (e.g., quality assurance)	Some will have formal business qualifications, sometime specifically in healthcare or primary care management. Most will have formal financial and HR training	
Pharmacist (Community or practice based) Increasingly involved in direct patient contact, quality assurance of prescribing, monitoring of long term and complex prescribing. Some (community) may be first point of contact for minor illness and advice, others (practice based) may have a more educational and supervisory role. They often have a key role in substance misuse services and may be qualified smoking counsellors	4-years masters degree and 1 year pre-registration in approved pharmacy	Varies. Some will have a lot of experience in organising placements and other training for staff and may have qualifications in adult education

(*Continued*)

(*Continued*)

Role	Training/career path (UK)	Educational involvement

Third sector/Voluntary sector

The third sector or voluntary sector is increasingly involved in the delivery of healthcare in all countries. Charities often employ specialist nurses and carers (e.g., cancer, heart disease, respiratory, dementia and mental health); their volunteers help support the PHCT in a variety of areas: e.g., palliative care, dementia care, supporting social needs such as housing and employment issues

There is a variety of set up from the informal involvement of the community, e.g., the community religious leaders, to the organised referral as part of specific pathways of care, e.g., McMillan nurses

Patient

The role of the patient is often said to be central to the work of the PHCT – however true patient-centred care empowers the patient to control the management. Many patients become expert in their own care and the diseases they have experienced – some even become experts in teaching students about them. Their role is considered in more depth later.

Learning with and from the primary healthcare team

Shadowing professionals

Shadowing involves learning and being led by an experienced professional; passive observation will be limited to just that, an 'experience'. Active learning involves more engagement. Ask yourself questions about the situations you encounter. In your team, what role is the professional playing? What are the strengths of this model of care? How would you communicate with this team member as a doctor? What would you be doing if you were in their place? What is the next move? What do you need to be better at in order to come out of the shadow and into independent practice?

TASK

Make sure you learn at least the following from members of the PHCT:
- How they were trained – for how long, based from where, what was involved?
- What professional development and accreditation do they have to complete?
- Who employs them?
- What their career progression looks like?

Every encounter with the PHCT will present you with an opportunity to learn from and about the bigger team. Even topics that are on the face of it purely 'medical' will have hidden facets that can deepen and reinforce your learning. One crucial area is learning about pharmacology, prescribing and therapeutics – often areas of concern to students (and crucial sources of error when considering patient safety). Spending time with the practice or community pharmacist and their team will not only enhance your understanding of their crucial role(s), but also help you learn both science and medicine.

Enhancing clinical skills and practical procedures

Working with the PHCT offers excellent opportunities to acquire or enhance clinical and procedural skills. Many of the basic clinical skills that medical students need to acquire are performed by members of the PHCT more often than by doctors. This includes communicating and explaining results of investigations; educating patients in tasks such as using inhalers and using contraception and many practical procedures from smear tests to phlebotomy. Practical skills, which you must learn in preparation for foundation year, are best learned with certain team members. Table 5.1 is based on the skills curriculum from one UK

Table 5.1 Clinical and procedural skills which could be perfected in community settings or with PHCT guidance. (Source: Barts and The London clinical skills curriculum)

	Year 1	Year 2	Year 3	Year 4	Year 5	PHCT taught?
Measuring body temperature (various ways)	O		O	O	O	GP/Nurse
Measuring radial pulse rate rhythm and character		O	O	O	O	GP/Nurse
Peripheral pulses, including anatomical locations			O	O	O	GP/Nurse
Blood pressure (manual and auto)	O	O	O	O	O	
Height and weight for adults and children	O	O	O	O	O	GP
Transcutaneous monitoring of O$_2$ sats			O	O	O	HCA, GP, nurse, midwife
Venepuncture with vacutainer system, sharps and clinical waste				O	O	
Management of blood samples	N/A					
Taking blood cultures	N/A					
Measuring blood glucose using reagent sticks with or without a glucometer			O		O	GP, Nurse, HCA
Managing an ECG monitor	N/A					
Performing and interpreting a 12 lead ECG			O	O	O	GP/Nurse/HCA
Basic respiratory function tests (Peak flow)			O	O	O	Nurse
Urinalysis using Multistix			O	O	O	Nurse/HCA
Advising patients on how to collect an MSU specimen			O	O	O	GP/Nurse/midwife
Taking nose, throat and skin swabs				O	O	GP/District Nurse
Nutritional assessment and interpretation of growth and BMI charts			O	O	O	GP/District Nurse/Health visitor
Pregnancy testing					O	GP/Nurse
Cervical smears and swabs					O	GP/Nurse
Administering oxygen			O		O	GP/District Nurse

Skill			
Establishing peripheral intravenous access and setting up an infusion; use of infusion devices	N/A*		
Making up drugs for parenteral administration	N/A		
Dosage and administration of insulin and use of sliding scales	N/A		
Using a nebulizer		○	
Insert a nasogastric tube	N/A*		
Subcutaneous and intramuscular injections		○	Both
Blood transfusion	N/A		
Male and female urinary catheterization	N/A*		
Radial Arterial Blood Gas Sample	N/A		
Instructing patients in the use of devices for inhaled medication (e.g., inhalers in asthma)		○	GP/Nurse
Use of local anaesthetics	N/A†		
Skin suturing	N/A†		
Order a blood transfusion	N/A		
Wound care and basic wound dressing		○	Nurse/District Nurse
First Aid, Control of haemorrhage		○	
Handwashing (6 steps). Scrub up and gown for sterile procedures	○	○	
Correct techniques for 'moving and handling', including patients		○	District Nurse
How to confirm death/ writing a death certificate		○	GP
'Basic Life Support' for adults and children		○	

Adapted from GMC (2009b) 'Tomorrow's Doctors' pp. 77–81.

*Although most appropriate for secondary care, placements may be taught whilst shadowing Specialist District Nurse Staff

†Although not available on all placements, minor surgery providers may optionally teach these skills

medical school and shows which may be best learned from PHCT members. In the United Kingdom, the list of the skills expected to be learned are outlined in appendix 1 to 'Tomorrow's doctors' (GMC, 2009b). You will find similar guidance from your own medical school and other national curricula. *Make sure you check your own expected learning outcomes, relevant to your own level of experience. If in doubt, discuss your needs with you placement tutor.*

Do not forget that the patient is central and that you are learning through the delivery of care to them. All members of the PHCT will respect your learning needs if you can reference them back to how they will help you help your patients in the future. Keep this in mind whether you are learning practical skills or skills for collecting and recording information. Most schools will insist (or should insist) on core competencies being signed off first in the clinical skills labs and away from patients. This may be worth mentioning to reassure those in the practice/ placement provider. This should also be clear in your procedural learning log/checklist/portfolio: do take these and share them with both your tutor and the various professionals who support your learning.

TIP

Identify specific learning outcomes each time you shadow a team member.

If you are timetabled to be with members of the PHCT make sure you check the objectives supplied as part of this; if in doubt ask your tutor what you should specifically try to get out of it.

Identify which, if any, particular clinical or procedural skills there may be a chance to develop or practice (and explore how this can best help the professional you are linked to – they may be delighted if you take blood samples or give injections, but do it only if you are competent to do so).

Learning from the practice nurses

Immunisation

In the United Kingdom, majority of immunisations are administered and organised by primary care nurses. Placements in general practice will give you opportunities to witness these immunisations being given and learn about the important contraindications and safety concerns. These will include children's vaccinations and also increasingly prevention of infection in vulnerable adults (e.g., those with long-term conditions, situations of immunosuppression or the elderly). Senior students may well be able to take part in the annual flu vaccination programme. You will be able to administer some injections after suitable training and under supervision.

TASK

Explore recent changes to the standard immunisation programmes.
What are the risk–benefits that clinicians need to consider before advising patients?
Discuss with the nurses and your tutor conflicting views about flu vaccinations.

Travel vaccination

Most UK travellers will seek advice about appropriate protection and vaccination prior to holidays and major trips abroad from the practice nurse. Most practices will provide standard travel vaccines (e.g., typhoid, hepatitis A and B and meningococcal protection). Some will provide additional specialist vaccinations for rabies or yellow fever. Tutorials about the subject, supplemented with practical sessions, will give you an opportunity to learn about the preparation of vaccines for administration and the details to be included in a consultation. Discussions about malaria prophylaxis could lead to shared learning with peers about world population health needs.

TASK

Identify the level of travel vaccination undertaken in your clinical placement.
   Discuss with the practice nurses where they get their vaccination guidance from.
   Determine how advice is offered about appropriate protection.
   Use your peer group to explore any additional information you need to provide that advice.

Learning from the pharmacy team

We explored in Chapter 1 how community placements can be ideal to consolidate learning about therapeutics and prescribing. Much of this learning will happen with the practice-based PHCT, either from practice-based pharmacists, community pharmacists or within consultations with members of the PHCT (e.g., practice nurses, nurse practitioners and of course GPs).

TASK: ACTIVE LEARNING WITH THE PHARMACY TEAM

Explore with your tutor the possibility of spending a half day with a community pharmacist (as well as with the practice pharmacist where you have one).

Start by asking them or finding out what their background is, how long the training was, who is their professional body, how are they reaccredited?

Make sure you *are actively involved* if possible with their work when you are with them; see if you can help explain to patients how to take their medication or contribute to giving advice on the common over the counter drugs that are given out. You'll soon learn the huge amount of healthcare happening outside of medical services in primary care, and the limits to your knowledge. Always ensure you are fully supervised. Keep a reflective diary of your experience, share it with colleagues.

Medicine-taking is a complex human behaviour and patients evaluate medicines and the risks and benefits of using medicines with the resources available to them. Unwanted and unused medicines reflect inadequate communication between professionals and patients – about health problems and how they might be treated, and about patients' ongoing assessment and experience of treatments. Practitioners have a duty to help patients make informed decisions about treatment and use

---

TIP

Always have an appropriate drug formulary such as the BNF in hand: hard copy or an App

Shadow prescribe drugs for every patient you see, look at the options and before long you will know what to prescribe, how much and how often!

appropriately prescribed medicines to best effect. Using a patient-centred approach to prescribing will ensure that patients views are included in the decision-making process and that suitable, accredited information about medicines is readily available from their practitioner.

While observing consultations you could decide to focus on the prescribing elements involved and consider some of the above issues. Was this done well? Did the patient understand the outcome for them? How sure are you that adherence will not be a problem? Reflect on the consultation and consider what aspects you can incorporate into your interactions with patients. In hospital settings, you are much less likely to see the whole process of prescribing through from clinical need and decision making to dispensing or even administration. In primary care or general practice you should take the chance and engage in this activity at all stages. It is fascinating and important.

TASK: GETTING ORIENTED, ACUTE PRESCRIBING

Ask your tutor if you could 'take the hot seat' and complete a consultation by handing over a prescription and explaining all aspects of the medication to the patient (what the medication is, how to take it, for how long and what to do if there are problems).

Ask your tutor when you see something prescribed, even an antibiotic, if you can 'follow the prescription' to the chemist, through any dispensing checks to any follow up checks and balances in the system to monitor drug usage [Acute prescribing]

Repeat prescribing

Almost all general practices in developed countries have systems for issuing repeat prescriptions to patients without the need for a consultation. In many countries, including the United Kingdom, the process is aided by clinical computer systems.

Receptionists and administrative staff make important 'hidden' contributions to quality and safety in repeat prescribing in general practice, regarding themselves accountable to patients for these contributions. Studying technology-supported work routines that seem mundane, standardised and automated, but which in reality require a high degree of local tailoring and judgement from frontline staff, opens up a new agenda for the study of patient safety (Swinglehurst *et al.*, 2011).

When qualified you will be responsible for any prescription you sign, including repeat prescriptions for medicines initiated by colleagues. As a doctor you must, therefore, make sure that any repeat prescription you sign is safe and appropriate. You should consider the benefits of prescribing repeats against the risks. At each review, you will need to confirm that the patient is taking their medicines as directed, and check that the medicines are still needed, effective and tolerated. This may be particularly important following a hospital stay, admission, appointment or home visit (GMC, 2013: Sections 55 and 58).

TASK: LEARNING ABOUT, AND FROM, REPEAT PRESCRIBING

Follow the 'repeat prescription request journey' for a patient taking multiple medicines.

Identify who makes decisions and what decisions are made regarding the issue of a particular medicine. Identify any risks that might be involved along that 'journey'. Identify what drugs might be less suitable for repeat prescribing systems and why. Who makes the decision and monitors changes?

Shadow the staff member arranging the issue of repeat prescriptions.

What steps are involved? Undertake an audit to identify how many medicines requested by patients as repeat items were missing from the repeat list. Identify the reasons for the discrepancies. How might these be reduced?

Prescribing in elderly patients and those with multiple long-term conditions

Note carefully the list of medications on repeat prescriptions for any patient over 75 years or any patient in long-term conditions clinics. The potential for confusion, error and drug interactions rise as the number of prescriptions rise – especially where they may be memory-related problems. Explore with your tutor and pharmacy team how such potential for error can be minimised and consider the task below to highlight the dangers and possible solutions.

TASK: PRESCRIBING HAZARDS IN MORE COMPLICATED PATIENTS

Ask your tutor to identify a patient with multiple long-term conditions. If possible arrange to visit them at home.

Explore with the patient their level of understanding of when and how they take their medicines and for what reason. Consider the clinical risks of any lack of understanding.

Explore where they keep their medicines. Are they up to date? Does the quantity match the record on the practice computer? Is there too little/much of one or more medicines? What does this say about usage and monitoring of repeat prescriptions?

Learning about adherence and patient safety issues

Barriers to medication adherence are complex and varied. A Medline literature review undertaken in 2010 is a good starting point to consider them (Brown and Bussell, 2011). There are many causes of non-adherence but they generally fall into two overlapping categories: intentional and unintentional.

Unintentional non-adherence occurs when the patient wants to follow the agreed treatment but is prevented from doing so by barriers beyond their control. Examples include poor recall or comprehension of instructions, difficulties in administering the treatment, inability to pay for the treatment or simply forgetting to take it. Unintentional non-adherence is related to limitations in the persons' capacity and resources affecting their ability to implement their intention to adhere.

TASK: ISSUES OF ADHERENCE

Ask your tutor to help identify a patient taking four or more regular medicines and undertake a 'Medication Review'/Medicines Use Review [MUR] with the patient, that is, discuss the use of the medicines and check that the patient understands the need for and mechanism of action of the medicines.

Identify any issues of non-adherence and why have they occurred.

• Consider what support the patient may need to improve adherence to treatment plans.

• Consider what strategies already exist to support the patient.

• Discuss with your peer group what processes might be utilised to improve the quality of prescribing and how waste of medicines in the NHS might be reduced.

Intentional non-adherence occurs when the person decides not to follow the treatment recommendations (NCCPC and RCGP, 2009). The above needs to be considered in the light of the WHO statement that increasing adherence may have a greater effect on health than any improvement in specific medical treatments (WHO, 2003).

There are many considerations involved in any prescribing decision, and many potential risks to patient safety. Any clinician prescribing for a patient's illness will need to be aware of any allergic response to a medicine or interactions with any other long-term medicine taken and ensure that the formulation is one which the patient can best use.

Access to community pharmacists will provide insight into their role in supporting patients in the safe and effective use of their medicines, together with providing education and increased understanding. The UK MUR scheme, provided by pharmacists, is designed to improve concordance and compliance by patients in the effective use of prescribed medications: http://psnc.org.uk/services-commissioning/advanced-services/murs/

CURIOSITIES: DISPENSING PRACTICES AND COMMUNITY PHARMACISTS

Patients that live in rural areas in the United Kingdom, and those who live more than 1 mile/1.6 km from a community pharmacy, can have their medicines dispensed from their GP surgery if those premises are registered as dispensing premises. Currently, there are 1086 dispensing practices in England which dispense to 3.34 million patients. (*Isom M. Dispense with Dependence. Management in Practice, 2013*). You might want to explore with your GP tutor and local community pharmacist, what the advantages and drawbacks of such a system are. Consider patient safety, prescribing error and patient convenience.

Roles of pharmacists, general practitioners and nurses in prescribing vary across countries. Ask locally about the situation – and its advantages and drawbacks for the patient and practitioner.

Primary health team meetings

Many practices will hold regular multidisciplinary team meetings where they share management of patients and co-ordinate management plans. Often these are within the practice-based teams and sometimes the wider community PHCT meetings. Usually they will be focussed around a particular area of care (e.g., palliative care review meetings for those with terminal illness) or a particular focus on quality governance (e.g., critical incident meetings). Explore with your tutor or administrative lead when these meetings are scheduled during your placement and which patients will be discussed. If possible try to see some of the patients or find out about their case from the notes. Contribute by asking questions about any aspects of case summaries that are not clear (if they are not clear to you as a fresh pair of eyes then it may not be clear to others and communication errors may result).

TASK: LEARNING FROM MULTIDISCIPLINARY TEAM (MDT) CASE DISCUSSIONS

Listen to the perspective brought by each member of the team; this is often apparent from the problems and issues that they raise and in the way each member contributes solutions.

Check with the clinicians involved first, but you could offer to contribute to patient care and see patients after such discussions. Often as a student you have more time and communicating the plan to the patient is a valuable skill to learn.

Ensure you write in your portfolio or reflective diary what you have learnt at these meetings. Remember to include your understanding of psychological and social aspects of the patients care as well as the medical management. Think about ethical and legal issues that arise (often around consent and competence) and about how resources are best used. Care plans often focus on overcoming barriers and setting goals. What examples have you seen?

Use these cases as examples if you have to write up a case for your medical school formative or summative assessment.

TASK: COMMUNICATION AND REFERRALS INTO THE PHCT

Ask your tutor if you could do the referral for a patient you have seen in the PHCT (e.g., to a podiatrist, physiotherapist or alternative practitioner or similar). Include information you have gathered from the patient, from the correspondence, from your own examination and the medical record. Put together your own assessment of the issue that you are writing to address. Suggest possible management and reference this to current guidelines. Don't forget to include what has already been tried, being done or planned.

Ask your tutor or the clinician involved to feedback on how complete your assessment is. Have you missed any information? Is the language you use and the management suggested appropriate? Such an exercise can often contribute considerably to the better care of the patient.

Always get your tutor to check the referral.

Learning from mistakes

The PHCT is a complex system and as with any organisation sometimes things go wrong. Regularly the team will review events or 'critical incidents' – where harm occurred or nearly occurred and the team as a whole as well as the individuals that make it up will reflect on these events. It is an explicit requirement of professional bodies for doctors to systematically review mistakes. For instance within the United Kingdom your revalidation as a doctor is subject to demonstrating participation in 'critical incident reviews'.

The Francis report (2013) records the UK public enquiry into deficient care at the Mid-Staffordshire NHS trust Hospital between 2005 and 2009. It recommends the introduction of a new statutory 'Duty of Candour' requiring all NHS staff and directors to be open and honest when mistakes happen. This places a legal obligation on health service provider organisations and individual practitioners to be honest, open and truthful in all their dealings with patients and the public.

You can learn about a number of important professional attitudes by taking part in this process. What kind of mistakes can happen? What problems in communication lead them to rise? How can the risk be reduced? What features of good teamwork can help? How are established practices changed? Your medical school may set learning tasks or case reports to cover this important professional principle – or you may be able to discuss it as a peer learning exercise.

Patients and public involvement in your education

You cannot learn to be a doctor by simply reading a text book. Patients are an essential part of clinical education. In primary care you will meet patients who often have the space and desire to communicate with you and contribute to your medical education. They are often less poorly, and so less passive, than in hospital settings – and perhaps therefore more forthcoming about their medical conditions, their carers and health professionals and their perspectives on ill-health.

The role of the patient within medicine has changed and continues to change – from a passive recipient of our 'care' to an increasingly active partner, indeed an expert, in their own health (Towle *et al.*, 2010). Research shows that such an approach benefits both the patients and the professionals; communication improves, patients are empowered to make behavioural changes and resources are better targeted to those that will use them (The Health Foundation, 2011). Patient interest groups have supported this shift in focus, whether to champion specific diseases or championing the role of the patient voice in improving healthcare, for example, The Picker institute (Picker Institute, 2015).

TASK

Consider a patient you have seen (choose one with your tutor) and try to consider their condition from the various perspectives of patient, carer, employer, GP, nurse etc. Then try to explore directly with these same people (including the patient) – what they think about their condition, how it affects their life, what the frustrations and fears are. How close were your ideas compared to the patients? How much did the patient's ideas differ from those of the professionals involved?

You may well have this or similar tasks to write up for your own medical school – we are not trying to duplicate work – but rather trying to suggest interesting and useful tasks to enhance understanding and learning.

Alongside the increased acceptance of patients as partners in healthcare, their role in medical education is rapidly changing. Medical schools and their governing bodies have to consider how to engage patients in teaching, curriculum design and assessment in a way that promotes partnership (Towle *et al.*, 2010). Examples include lay representation on interview panels to a compulsory patient feedback as part of licensing (such as revalidation in the United Kingdom). Some work explores how this relates to primary care teaching practices (e.g., Lucas and Pearson, 2012).

Patients are generally well informed and are experts of their own conditions. They are therefore well placed both to help you inform about their condition and also help you appreciate the patient perspective. This is essential when having discussions with patients about treatment decisions and to ensure joint understanding and ownership of the management plan (and improve adherence to agreed treatment plans). Involvement of patients in your learning may be on a one-to-one basis or as part of a small group teaching. Think what patients may be able to teach you beyond practising how to take history or perform an examination. Patients come to see their GP with diverse presentations of common conditions. How, when and why patients present are questions that you should ask of yourself and patients.

Patients are encouraged to comment on the quality of care and service provided to them and doctors are required to reflect on the survey results of patient opinion as a requirement for revalidation. Most patients are keen to be involved in student education and increasingly there is a need for you as students to hear feedback from them, either directly or indirectly via your tutor. Indeed in the United Kingdom the GMC suggests 'Ensure that you seek feedback about your performance from patients or carers after contact with a patient in a learning setting' (GMC, 2009a; Para 111).

You will meet and learn from patients and the public in a variety of ways:
- Current patients attending clinics
- Carers, advocates and support workers
- 'Expert' patients (real patients with training to enhance their role in education)
- Simulated patients (actors or role-players)
- Virtual patients (often developed with input from 'real' patients)
- Lay teachers (often chosen because of relevant expertise)
- Patient groups and representatives (either based on a particular service or location)
- Local and National community and third sector organizations

(UK GMC (2009c) Supplementary Guidance to Tomorrow's Doctors 'Patient and Public involvement in Undergraduate Medical Education')

All UK general practices are now required to have a 'Patient Participation Group'. These groups allow registered patients of a practice to comment on changes proposed in the practice, general concerns raised by patients or on the results of the annual patient survey. This can be a positive mechanism to input ideas for service developments for the practice to consider. Attending one of these groups will provide a valuable insight into what patients value from their doctors and nurses.

TASK: PATIENT INVOLVEMENT WITH EDUCATION IN THE PRACTICE

Explore with the practice manager or equivalent how the practice/organisation uses patient feedback; do they collect it?

Arrange to meet/attend the practice's patient participation group while in placement. Explore how the patient's opinion is included in decisions about the service provided. What effect have recent initiatives had on patients' well-being?

Ask your tutor how the practice involves patients in teaching. How are they asked? What benefits do they get? How do they feedback on the students and on their experience?

Summary

Chapter 5 has explored how best to learn from the primary health care team, especially those colleagues in the practice or health centre where you will spend the majority of your placements. We hope the advice offered will help you achieve two things. The first to find out more about the roles, skills and training of various members of the clinical team and the second to use their expertise and experience to gain knowledge, skills and attitudes which will be essential to make you better clinicians.

References

Brown MT, Bussell JK (2011) Medication adherence: WHO cares? Mayo Clinic Proceedings 86 (4): 304–314.

CANMEDS Family Medicine Working Group on Curriculum Review October 2009, College of Family Physicians of Canada accessed at www.cfpc.ca. Accessed 15 July 2015.

Francis R (2013) Report of the Mid Staffordshire NHS Foundation Trust Public Inquiry: Executive Summary. London: Stationery Office.

GMC (2009a) Tomorrow's Doctors. General Medical Council of UK. www.gmc-uk.org. Accessed 15 July 2015.

GMC (2009b) Appendix 1 to Tomorrow's Doctors especially page 79–81 for practical skills. www.gmc-uk.org. Accessed 15 July 2015.

GMC (2009c) Patient and public involvement in undergraduate medical education Advice supplementary to *Tomorrow's Doctors* (2009) General Medical Council of UK. www.gmc-uk.org. Accessed 15 July 2015.

GMC (2013) Good practice in prescribing and managing medicines and devices. Sections 55 and 58. General Medical Council of UK. www.gmc-uk.org. Accessed 15 July 2015.

Lucas B, Pearson D (2012) Patient perceptions of their role in undergraduate medical education within a primary care teaching practice. Education for Primary Care 23: 277–285.

NCCPC and RCGP (2009) Medicines Adherence: involving patients in decisions about prescribed medicines and supporting adherence. Available http://www.nice.org.uk/nicemedia/pdf/cg76fullguideline.pdf. Accessed 15 July 2015.

Picker Institute (2015) http://www.pickereurope.org/about-us/. Accessed 15 July 2015.

Swinglehurst D, Greenhalgh T, Russell J, Myall M (2011) Receptionist input to quality and safety in repeat prescribing in UK general practice: ethnographic case study. BMJ 343: Article d6788.

The Health Foundation (2011) Helping people to help themselves: a review of the evidence considering whether it is worthwhile to support self-management. Available at http://www.health.org.uk/publication/evidence-helping-people-help-themselves. Accessed 15 July 2015.

Towle A, Bainbridge L, Godolphin W, Katz A, Kline C, Lown B, Madularu I, Solomon P, Thistlethwaite J (2010) Active patient involvement in the education of health professionals. Medical Education 44 (1): 64–74.

WHO (2003) Adherence to Long-term Therapies: Evidence for Action. Geneva, Switzerland: World Health Organisation.

Further resources

CAIPE (centre for the advancement of interprofessional education) has much on multi and interprofessional working and learning. www.caipe.org.uk. Accessed 15 July 2015.

CANMEDS Family Medicine Working Group on Curriculum Review October 2009, College of Family Physicians of Canada provides a good example of mapping a general competency framework to community (family) practice. www.cfpc.ca. Accessed 15 July 2015.

HealthWatch UK. www.healthwatch.co.uk. Accessed 15 July 2015.

National Association of Patient Participation in Primary Care (UK). http://www.napp.org.uk/index.html. Accessed 15 July 2015.

Chapter 6 Learning medicine in community settings

With Ann O'Brien and Will Spiring

One of the great privileges of community placements is the chance to see how patients live their lives and, at first hand, the impact of those lifestyles on their health and their ill health on their lives. The great majority of healthcare occurs in the community, and often outside of health centres and general practice surgeries. For the most poorly or disabled patients, care may be within their own home or residential homes.

This chapter will address the nature and benefits of learning from a range of community settings, including the wider community healthcare team. We will explore a little the way care is provided in community settings, but concentrate mainly on what opportunities there are to learn medicine and how you can maximise this on your placements.

For many reasons doctors do fewer 'home visits' than some years ago and often these are restricted to palliative care visits. There is however a wide range of other health professional from whom you can learn during their visits, for example, mental health teams, women and children's services, district nurses, specialist community nurses and palliative care teams.

By the end of this chapter you should be able to:

- to further understand the impact of ill-health on patients' lives and approaches taken to deal with it
- understand which healthcare services are delivered in the community, in patient's homes or places of residence

How to Succeed on Primary Care and Community Placements, First Edition.
David Pearson and Sandra Nicholson.
© 2016 John Wiley & Sons, Ltd. Published 2016 by John Wiley & Sons, Ltd.

- understand the roles of the teams delivering community-based healthcare and their interaction.
- appreciate how visits to patients' homes can strengthen the understanding of clinicians and support the delivery of healthcare for the most vulnerable patients.

Learning from community visits

Within the United Kingdom there has been a recent drive to increase the provision of 'care closer to home' with a wide variety of health-related services, now commonly community based (DH; Transforming Community Settings; Ambitions, Action, Achievement, 2009). This document outlines how further aspects of the acute care of patients, as well as patients' ongoing care are to be provided within local community services. As medical students it is important that you learn how 'care closer to home' involves a variety of allied health professionals, such as pharmacists, community mental health teams and children's services (e.g., Sure Start in the United Kingdom). They all provide an increasing number of support initiatives closer to the patients' homes. The community visits you undertake while on your placement may involve a variety of settings including patients' homes, child centres, outreach clinics and residential or nursing homes.

There are a large number of services commonly delivered in community settings. All of these provide opportunities for you to meet patients. The various health professionals will work closely with each other to deliver care in or close to the patients' homes. They will be involved with patients from 'cradle to grave'. Students will be able to witness patients at various points in their journeys along the pathway of their illness and you are encouraged to take advantage of the learning opportunities available. There are other services that might be variably available in different parts of the country, depending on local commissioning decisions of health boards. These might include domiciliary physiotherapy providing treatment for chronic lung disease, acute or chronic locomotor or neurological problems to aid rehabilitation.

As a starting point to understand the complexity of health and social care in the community, consider the following task with your tutor:

TASK

Ask your tutor to help identify a housebound patient with a long-term neurological problem.

Explore, from the care record, the background and nature of the problems the patient faces.

Arrange to visit the patient (ideally with your tutor or a specialist nurse) and explore the input of therapy services and level of rehabilitation achieved.

Explore the patient's perspective of their health status and the care they receive.

What adaptations have been made to help the patient and their care(s) to manage at home?

Learning from doctor's home visits

The nature and complexity of the medical needs of patients have changed so significantly over the past few years, together with greater transport availability for the majority in the United Kingdom, that home visits are now almost exclusively undertaken for the housebound.

Historically, the impression of a traditional doctor in the United Kingdom is the 'doctor doing his rounds' which was embedded in his usual practice. He (usually 'he'!) would be a member of the community that all would know and trust. One unique remaining feature of general practice is the opportunity (sometimes the expectation) of seeing patients in their own home. Home is where patients generally feel safest. Inclusion of an assessment of the living environment may often offer insight and a wider recognition of barriers to effective care delivery. There is good evidence that home visits for elderly housebound patients reduce mortality and nursing home admissions (Elkan, 2001). A recent meta-analysis of trials supports the hypothesis that preventive home visitation programmes are effective in delaying functional decline in elderly patients, mortality and nursing home admissions (Stuck *et al.*, 2002).

The medical needs of patients requiring a home visit tend to be more complex as such patients usually have multiple morbidity and complex social needs – whether for physical or mental reasons. Visiting patients in their own homes therefore provides rich learning opportunities for you to appreciate how patients cope with the practical issues of living with disability and long-term conditions.

> **TASK**
>
> It is likely that your medical school will encourage you to visit a housebound patient or one with multiple long-term conditions in their own home.
>   Consider what you are being asked to do and how that opportunity will help you meet those objectives.
>   Discuss it and agree a realistic outcome with your tutor.
>   Who looks after the medical needs? How many individuals are involved? What do they do? How co-ordinated are their interventions?

The carers of such patients may also be burdened by their role and will need consideration in any care discussions. These issues are important for you to consider when you draw up management plans and evaluate patient adherence with medication. Equally these patients are the ones most dependant on a well-functioning community healthcare team.

> **TASK**
>
> Visiting patients at home is not as much a feature of general practice than it was 25 years ago. It is almost unheard of in many countries.
>   Discuss with your tutor the pros and cons of home visiting:
> • Which patients are seen? How has this changed over time?
> • What are the problems caused by home visits?
> • What are the issues over patient safety and the safety of clinical staff?
> • How is data entered into patient records?

Visiting patients in their own homes and reviewing their care plans provides opportunities for you to learn how multidimensional assessments and frequent follow up has now become part of the strategies for the Clinical Commissioning Groups for the delivery of Integrated Care arrangements within England and Wales. These strategies aim to reduce unplanned and avoidable admissions through the Accident and Emergency departments (NHS Institute for Innovation and Improvement, 2008).

Choosing from one of the following tasks to help you explore how patients cope with their long-term health conditions while in their own homes and how health professional seek to reduce emergency admissions will facilitate your learning.

TASK

Visit an identified patient who has had frequent hospital admissions.

Learn about what interventions have been put in place to help the patient remain in their own home. Which health professionals were involved? Consider how this activity will help you learn about initiatives to look after patients at home.

Interview a patient who has had a recent admission to hospital and is identified to be at risk of more (your tutor or the practice manager will help!). Explore the practical problems that the admission might cause, for example, caring roles of others, pet care, regular deliveries, etc. How were these resolved previously?

Visiting residential care and nursing homes

I found it useful that there was such a variety of experience, for instance we visited both the caring and nursing homes to view community care from another angle

(Medical Student on Year 5 Community Care Module)

Some patients, whether old or young, require more assistance than others and in these instances their home is often within the institutional care system. Irrespective of the type of residence, all patients need access to general primary care. Residential care can offer a range of support from general care and nutrition support to twenty-four hour board and nursing care support.

Patients who move from their own homes to become residents of permanent care will have diverse backgrounds, needs and aspirations for their care. They will be a rich source of life experience and generally be pleased to support your learning by sharing that experience with you. Residents of care homes and nursing homes within the United Kingdom will be registered with a local GP who is responsible for their medical care. These patients will often be vulnerable for a variety of reasons – multiple pathology, multiple medications, possibly poor memory and poor mobility. Excellent clinical skills are needed to diagnose conditions in patients who may be unable to communicate completely. Some will have been admitted because of the necessity of care needs and others will become residents because of social isolation or risk, perhaps not from personal choice. Many GP surgeries have specific responsibilities for individual homes.

Visit a nursing home and observe the strategies involved in caring for vulnerable adults who cannot communicate for themselves. Investigate the legal responsibilities and requirements involved when caring for these people. In particular your community placements are opportunities for you to gain an understanding of the principles and practices concerning safeguarding vulnerable adults, assessing capacity and issues to do with consent covered by the Care Act (2014) (Geriatrics Society, 2009; Boland *et al.*, 2013).

As institutional care is expensive, there are financial and wider social imperatives to prevent ill-health and increasing disability in the elderly, thus enabling them to remain independent and in their own homes for as long as possible. Potential savings to the Medicaid programme, from using Home and Community-Based Services rather than institutional care, could be $57 338 for each participant in 2006 – national savings of $57 billion (Harrington *et al.*, 2011).

TASK: LEARNING FROM RESIDENTIAL HOME VISITS

On residential home visits within your community placements we suggest you concentrate on those aspects of medicine and care you can best learn in this setting. Many medical schools will have already a specified set of learning objectives such as the following:

- What are the patient's own perspectives of their problems?
- Who cares for them? Who provides their basic human needs, which are more important than medical ones – food, warmth, security, love, faith?
- Consider the health and social needs of the individual within the context of why they came to live here?
- How do multiple staff and healthcare professionals interact to optimally provide care?

Learning from community mental health teams

Drug and alcohol services

Approaches to the support of individuals with drug and alcohol dependency are mainly delivered through community-based services. The skills required to support these individuals are broad and varied. There is often the need to consider the impact of these behaviours on family members, especially children. Staff in drug misuse services, in key working or similar roles could be involved in the provision of low-intensity psychosocial interventions both for drug-specific interventions and for common mental disorders. For some staff, this will already form a key element of their roles and duties (e.g., motivational interviewing, which is a skilled form of patient–healthcare professional interaction used to encourage behavioural change).

Some services may expect all staff to deliver low-intensity interventions, and in others a phased approach to the delivery of these interventions may be developed. In still others, only certain groups may deliver some or all of the low-intensity interventions (National Treatment Agency for Substance Misuse, 2010).

It has been estimated that roughly 13% of Australian children live in a home with at least one adult who misuses alcohol (Dawe *et al.*, 2007). The Australian government has produced a resource sheet that discusses

Case Study

'Managing an addiction and keeping a family together can be a struggle'.

Through our drug and alcohol services we have been able to help people like Jim and his family to regain each other's trust and rebuild their relationships. Jim's key worker has helped him connect with his children again.

When Jim was at his lowest point he wasn't able to cope with his addiction or with being a parent. Jim's key worker, Natalie, quickly arranged for his two young children to be looked after by their older sister – an option that was far better than having them put into foster care. She referred him to a specialist structured day programme for people with substance misuse problems, where he also stayed as an inpatient.

His children in the meantime were safe and with this in mind he had time to get better without the added pressure of making sure they were looked after. Even after Jim finished his treatment, Natalie continued to keep in regular contact with the children's social worker and their school to keep them up to date with Jim's progress. Managing an addiction and keeping a family together can b e a struggle, but during regular key working sessions, Natalie and Jim came up with techniques to help him manage at home as well.

http://www.hestia.org/domestic-abuse/drugs-alcohol-/

> **TASK**
>
> Find out what local services are available and choose to spend a half-day visiting the facility, talk with local drug and alcohol rehabilitation workers and consider the impact of these problems on two patients with different backgrounds.
> Discuss the roles undertaken with the different drug & alcohol staff and the skills needed to achieve those roles.
> Meet a patient who has or has had a drug and/or alcohol dependency and explore the triggers for substance misuse behaviours.
> Explore the impact on any family members.
> Reflect on which of the learning objectives this activity has met.

guidelines on alcohol consumption, the effects of alcohol on parenting behaviour and the relationship between alcohol abuse and child maltreatment (Australian Institute of Family Studies, 2011).

Drug misusers, especially those with severe dependency, will often have many other problems. These include involvement with the criminal justice system, poor educational and employment histories, mental health issues, family problems and housing needs. Many have poor social and personal resources upon which to build a new life. Local partnerships to develop comprehensive and multidisciplinary systems have been shown to enable drug misusers to build a lifestyle that promotes health and well-being, social and personal capital, as well as tackling drug dependence.

Integrating robust pathways with employment services is a priority. Additionally solid partnership arrangements that support the families of drug misusers are also required. Developing mutual aid networks may help to establish self-help arrangements among recovering drug misusers (NHS National Treatment Agency for Substance Misuse, 2009).

> **TASK**
>
> You may consider working with the practice manager or admin lead to explore 'the prevalence of drug/alcohol etc. in the practice' and reflect on how difficult it might be to get this data. This would be a good topic for an SSC or as a peer group activity for discussion. *If in doubt ask your tutor.*
> Discuss interventions used by one or two patients and the evidence of success in achieving health and well-being.

Long-term mental healthcare in the community

Most mental healthcare is now managed in the community, with psychiatric hospital services reserved for the acute exacerbations of long-term conditions (acute psychosis, mania and the like). At best your medical school will have integrated mental health placements, with links to both acute and community services and opportunities to engage with community psychiatric nurses and others in the team (social workers, councillors etc.). You will also see a huge amount of mental ill health within routine primary care and general practice, with most stable conditions managed by GPs.

TASK

Ask your tutor to arrange to discuss with a patient with an enduring mental illness how they manage their condition within the community:
- What services do they access?
- Which healthcare professionals do they engage with?
- How are their medicines administered?
- What support can they access if they feel unwell.
- What is the balance between community and hospital services?

Many physical illnesses have an element of mental health overlay such as anxiety, depression, confused state or altered help-seeking behaviour. As healthcare practitioners we should be alert to this and where appropriate screen for it. Do not forget that patients with learning difficulties will sometimes express mental ill health alongside their physical needs.

If you have a particular interest in mental illness and psychiatry you will be able to focus on these aspects of routine surgeries, plus seek additional experiences with community mental health teams.

All medical students should at least learn to appreciate the importance of considering the psychosociol aspects alongside the physical when formulating care and management plans.

TASK

Arrange with your tutor to visit, in pairs or as a small group, a community hostel for residents with learning difficulties and/or long-term mental health problems.

Talk to the residents and explore the background to their world.
Consider what triggers have existed to cause their illness.
Discuss with your peers and tutor the psychosocial aspects for these residents.
Consider when early interventions might produce improved outcomes.

Community mental health for the elderly

Changing demographics across the world and rapidly increasing life expectancies are leading to a predicted significant rise in the survival of elderly and very elderly patients. Alongside this is an associated increase in a variety of long-term mental health problems, both depression and anxiety linked to long-term medical conditions and social isolation, and also a rise in dementia as a primary disease (Alzheimer's and associated dementias) or secondary to the same long-term conditions (cardiovascular disease and Parkinson's disease to name but two). Such mental health problems complicate medical and social care provision in the community and will impact on all of us as clinicians in the future (being equally important to the surgeon wanting to plan day treatments, as for the GP having to advise on fitness to drive and competency issues). Your primary care and community placements will give you the chance to learn from community mental health teams and the voluntary sector (e.g., MIND, Parkinson's disease societies etc.) to see how patients have their independence prolonged and care given with safety and dignity.

The number of people living with dementia in the United Kingdom alone is now close to 850 000, rising to one million by 2025. In the United Kingdom, the financial burden is £26.3 billion with costs attributable to both public and privately funded health and social care and informal care (Alzheimers Society, 2014). A skilled workforce of the future will be required to provide high-quality care within a few years. You will be that workforce! The multifaceted aspects of care of the dementia sufferer will provide you an unparalleled opportunity to consider not only the essentials of physical healthcare, but person-centred dementia care in collaboration with the multidisciplinary teams and voluntary organisations.

Learning to recognise dementia early and discussing issues of cultural diversity for dementia patients is only really possible by seeing patients in the primary care setting. Dementia UK supports local Admiral Nursing teams who provide practical and emotional support to family carers (http://www.dementiauk.org/what-we-do/admiral-nurses/).

Organise to attend a local day hospital and learn from the staff and patients what behaviours and attitudes are needed to support the care of dementia patients. Discuss what you learned with your peers or write up a case study for your portfolio. Do not miss the opportunity!

TASK

Identify, with your tutor, a patient with memory problems.

Explore with a patient and their carer(s) the problems they face and the impact on their lives and families.

Review the different health professionals that provide support for patients with memory problems.

If possible attend an appointment with a patient at their memory clinic.

Community maternity and child health services

Pregnancy, childbirth and early newborn care

Another great strength of community placements is that they allow an appreciation of the care of women during pregnancy and childbirth. Most pregnant mothers are healthy, and their antenatal and increasingly their perinatal and postnatal care are confined exclusively to community health professionals (midwives and specialist midwives). It is much easier to appreciate the scientific, social, psychological and medical aspects of pregnancy by learning from patients in community settings. Such encounters are more powerful when part of longitudinal integrated placements, where a pregnancy can be followed up to and after the birth. Some medical schools' curricula are designed to ensure students have such opportunities and all community placements provide good learning experiences regarding pregnancy, routine antenatal care, perinatal care for new mothers and their babies just following birth and

TASK

Review the different health professionals that provide support for women in the community during and immediately after pregnancy.

Ask your tutor if you can shadow one of the health professionals involved during a day's work. Make sure you are given some specific objectives for the day, which should include identifying the nature, extent and limits to their work.

then leading on to the first year of life. Such learning opportunities are usually provided by healthcare professionals other than GPs, midwives and health visitors, and so again we encourage you to learn from other professions and understand how optimal healthcare is integrated.

Children's services in the community

Most healthcare contacts with preschool children occur either within community health centres with health visitors or at the GP surgery. In addition many parents get considerable support from local children's community facilities, for example, Sure Start (United Kingdom). Use your time on community placements to talk with parents with young children about their fears, how they cope with minor illnesses and work commitments, who they get advice and support from and where health professionals fit into this. Use the placement to interact with children of different ages to experience the normal developmental milestones of young children. Attendance at the child health surveillance clinics will support this learning. You may also get the chance to spend time with children who are particularly dependant, vulnerable or have special educational needs or disabilities. Engaging with such opportunities can be a rewarding educational experience, especially if you have a particular interest in child health. Ask your tutor if you are interested.

> **TASK**
>
> Arrange to spend time at a community facility for preschool children.
> - Explore parental concerns, and the part the centre plays in their lives and how it contributes to supporting their family.
> - Refer the work by Joe Kai and others about parental fears of fever and see if the parents you met had the same worries (Kai, 1996; Crocetti *et al.*, 2001).
> - Use opportunities to play with young children of different ages.
> - Help health professionals assess and plot developmental milestones.
> - Discuss with health visitors their role and how it is changing.

Community sexual health services

Many sexual health treatment and screening services are provided in the community by specialist nurses. Some provision is provided in the surgery (especially near-patient testing, e.g., Chlamydia testing and screening).

A great many consultations revolve around anxieties related to sexual infections or contacts, so many common concerns affecting genitalia are discussed and treated appropriately before specialist services are involved (e.g., candidiasis, eczema, lichen planus, psoriasis). You will learn to identify occasions when sensitivity and non-judgemental communication skills are needed, plus having the chance to observe issues of consent and confidentiality.

You will also get the opportunity to see a range of contraceptive services and the preparation and counselling for these – both in the surgery but often in family planning clinics. Counselling for unwanted pregnancies usually occurs initially in general practice. These are not straightforward. Take the opportunities to observe and learn about this when on placement.

Placements where the focus of learning is women's health will also have ideal situations to consider all aspects of gynaecological conditions, whether that be practicing asking those intimate questions or undertaking sensitive examinations. It is important to remember though that some women will be reluctant to be examined by male students, and this choice needs to be accepted gracefully, however frustrating it must be.

TASK

Ask your tutor to spend time with sexual health or family planning services (whether practice based or community based)

- Identify where those concerned about sexual health seek advice, and why they choose a particular service.
- Explore with health professionals how they seek to improve access and preserve confidentiality.
- Explore issues of data recording, contact tracing and confidentiality, especially in cases of HIV or Hepatitis B & C.
- Familiarise yourself with near patient testing, screening and prevention programmes (e.g., HPV and Chlamydia).
- Are specific services available or provision made for high risk or hard to reach groups?

Palliative and end of life care

Most patients with cancer and other terminal illnesses are cared for in the community, albeit with crucial interventions by highly skilled specialist teams (e.g., palliative radiotherapy and chemotherapy units). Such care may be provided by the regular primary healthcare team in the practice or community or by specialist nurses (e.g., Macmillan, Marie Curie or local hospice outreach services and specialist pain nurses). We will explore what you can learn from these patients and their professional carers within your community placement, but obviously this will depend on you clearly identifying with your medical school or tutor what learning objectives there are for this topic.

When there is no cure for an illness, palliative care tries to make the end of a person's life as comfortable as possible. This is done by providing psychological, social and spiritual support together with clinical interventions to relieve pain and symptomatic suffering. Primary care will offer carers and family emotional support also as part of this 'holistic' approach to care (available at: http://www.nhs.uk/CarersDirect/guide/bereavement/Pages/Accessingpalliativecare.aspx)

Palliative care can be offered following treatments for cancer or in end stage long-term chronic diseases, such as COPD or chronic heart failure. This can be particularly important for children and young people who may live with a life-limiting condition for a long time.

Patients can receive palliative care in one, or often more than one, of the following:
- own home, hospice or residential home;
- day patient in a hospice, or
- hospital/specialist care

The provision of care and support in these situations is provided by the GP, district nurses, community palliative care nurses, such as Macmillan nurses, counsellors and social services. When care is provided at home, the GP is generally the named co-ordinator of care. The role of the named co-ordinator is paramount to facilitate communication between the key healthcare professionals. This co-ordinating role is now embedded within the practice approach to palliative care. The number and specialisation of professionals involved will vary according to the needs of the patient and their family. The integration of care achieved by effective teamwork across health, social services and hospice care ultimately improves outcomes for patients and families. UK End of Life Care has been influenced by an evidence-based approach intended to encourage this integration. These *Gold Standard Framework* and *One Chance to Get It Right* (Leadership

Alliance for the Care of Dying People, 2014) recommendations ensure a comprehensive approach to palliative care. It is worth exploring these with your tutor or the specialist nurses on your placements. Take the chance to learn about end of life decision making including pain control, palliative drug use, 'Do Not Resuscitate' guidance and ultimately after death regulations and requirements. Refer back to Chapter 5.

TASK

Ask your tutor to help identify a patient with a terminal illness and arrange to meet him/her to explore their experiences, their condition and the support and care received.

Ask your tutor to arrange for you to meet the community palliative care team and explore their role in the care of the identified patient. Use the learning objectives of your curriculum to identify areas for discussion.

Consider the importance of non-healthcare support in the patients you see. Take into consideration both the essential input of family and carers and also from the voluntary sector workers, faith groups or complimentary medicine input.

The holistic role of general practitioners is valued by patients and their families, in particular at the time of bereavement. Contact with funeral directors can be arranged by community care tutors. Spending a few hours with them may appear macabre, but will offer a fascinating insight into this important part of the wider community care team. It is important for tomorrow's doctors to understand the legal aspects governing the completion of death certificates and authorisation for cremation forms. You may wish to discuss with your tutor or peers the legal aspects of death certification and referrals to the coroner in situations of sudden death. Finally, if you are particularly interested in palliative and end of life care you could organise an elective or undertake a Student Selected Placement working at a hospice and with community palliative care specialists.

TASK

Arrange to visit the local coroner's office.

Discuss how a death is certified after postmortem.

Explore what the legal requirements of health professionals are?

Try and see examples of good and poor death certification.

Summary

This chapter has emphasised some of the truly unique opportunities to learn from patients, their carers and those that provide healthcare services, within the context of a patient's home and community. It is a real privilege to be welcomed into patients' homes and trusted with the details of their personal and social lives, as well as the medical information you get more readily in other settings. We have explained how through a range of interactions with a variety of health professionals, you can learn more about what makes multi-disciplinary team care effective. In addition we have illustrated how community placements encourage you to gain a better insight into the variety of community-based services that form essential services for many of our most vulnerable patients.

References

Alzheimers Society (2014) Available at http://www.alzheimers.org.uk/site/scripts/documents_info.php?documentID=341. Accessed 16 March 2015.

Australian Institute of Family Studies (2011) Alcohol Misuse and Child Maltreatment. ISSN 1448-9112 (Online). Available at http://www.aifs.gov.au/nch/pubs/sheets/rs27/index.html. Accessed 6 July 2015.

Boland B, Burnage J, Chowhan H (2013) Safeguarding adults at risk of harm. BMJ 14(346):f2716.

Crocetti M, Moghbeli N, Serwint J (2001) Fever phobia revisited: have parental misconceptions about fever changed in 20 years? Pediatrics 107(6):1241–1246.

Dawe S, Frye S, Best D, Moss D, Atkinson J, Evans C, Lynch M, Harnett P (2007) *Drug Use in the Family: Impacts and Implications for Children*, ANCD Research Paper; 13, report prepared for Australian National Council on Drugs, Canberra, ACT. Report available from: http://www.ancd.org.au/Publications-and-Reports/research-papers.html. Accessed 15 July 2015.

DH; Transforming Community Settings; Ambitions, Action, Achievement Jun 2009. Available at https://www.gov.uk/government/uploads/system/uploads/attachment_data/file/215781/dh_124196.pdf. Accessed 6 July 2015.

Elkan R (2001) Effectiveness of home based support for older people: systematic review and meta-analysis. BMJ. 323(7315):719–725.

Harrington C, Ng T, Kitchener M (2011) Do Medicaid home and community based service waivers save money? Home Health Care Services Quarterly Oct 30(4):198–213.

Kai J (1996) What worries parents when their preschool children are acutely ill, and why: a qualitative study. BMJ 313:983.

Leadership Alliance for the Care of Dying People (2014) Gold Standard Framework and One Chance to Get It Right (Leadership Alliance for the Care of Dying People; June 2014). Leadership Alliance etc: http://goldstandardsframework.org.uk/leadership-alliance-for-the-care-of-dying-people-lacdp. Accessed 7 July 2015. One Chance to Get it Right: https://www.gov.uk/government/uploads/system/uploads/attachment_data/file/323188/One_chance_to_get_it_right.pdf. Accessed 7 July 2015.

National Treatment Agency for Substance Misuse (2010) Routes to Recovery: Psychosocial Interventions for Drug Misuse. A framework and toolkit for implementing NICE-recommended treatment interventions. http://www.nta.nhs.uk/uploads/psychosocial_toolkit_june10.pdf. Accessed 19 November 2013.

NHS Institute for Innovation and Improvement (2008) Demand Management. Available at http://www.institute.nhs.uk/quality_and_service_improvement_tools/quality_and_service_improvement_tools/demand_and_capacity_-_demand_management.html. Accessed 6 July 2015.

NHS National Treatment Agency for Substance Misuse (2009) Commissioning for Recovery: Drug treatment, Reintegration and Recovery in the Community and Prisons. Guidance notes on completion of 2010/11 plans for drug partnerships. http://www.nta.nhs.uk/uploads/treatment_plan_guidance_2010_11.pdf. Accessed 7 July 2015.

Safeguarding Vulnerable Older People (Abuse and Neglect) - Best Practice Guide; British Geriatrics Society (2009) http://www.bgs.org.uk/index.php/topresources/publicationfind/goodpractice/88-safeguarding-vulnerable-older-people-abuse-and-neglect. Accessed 7 July 2015.

Stuck EA, Eggar M, Hammer A, Minder C, Beck JC (2002) Home visits to prevent nursing home admission and functional decline in elderly people: systematic review and meta-regression analysis. JAMA 287(8):1022–1028.

UK Gov. Care Act 2014. Published by TSO (The Stationary Office) Norwich, UK. Available at: http://www.legislation.gov.uk/ukpga/2014/23/pdfs/ukpga_20140023_en.pdf. Accessed 7 July 2015.

Further resources

NHS Choices/End of Life Care (2015) http://www.nhs.uk/Planners/end-of-life-care/Pages/what-is-end-of-life-care.aspx. 15 July 2015.

Sarna R, Thompson R (2008) Admiral nurses' role in a dementia carers' information programme. Nursing Older People 20(9), 30–34.

Chapter 7 **Clinical information systems, opportunities to learn**

With Jane Kirby

This chapter aims to stimulate learning with and about the clinical information systems which are an integral feature of patient care, especially in UK general practice. We believe that understanding the scope of what these systems offer and how they support patient care is core to your learning (Tomorrow's Doctors TD19 a-e; GMC, 2009). More importantly we believe they can help support your learning (as they still support ours as practicing clinicians).

By the end of this chapter you should be able to:

- understand what a clinical information system(CIS) is
- appreciate how a CIS integrates and improves a patient's care
- engage with a CIS to facilitate your learning
- safely use CISs and patient information
- learn the importance of Read codes and how to accurately use them

What are clinical information systems?

A clinical information system (CIS)…

> … is typically a computerised medical record that provides the usual functions of the patient's paper record.
>
> It enables the recording of clinical data generated at times of patient-professional interaction and the presentation of such data at subsequent contacts.

How to Succeed on Primary Care and Community Placements, First Edition.
David Pearson and Sandra Nicholson.
© 2016 John Wiley & Sons, Ltd. Published 2016 by John Wiley & Sons, Ltd.

Clinical data include problems, symptoms, signs, diagnoses, severity scales, patient expectations, plans, medication, interventions and outcomes.

UK Select Committee of Health (2007)

A clinical information system (CIS) supports and enhances the patient's electronic record – like MS Word is to your saved documents or your Computer Operating System is to your filed digital photos. It is the system that allows you to view all the saved data about a patient in one place.

Why learn about clinical information systems?

At present one of the great differences you'll notice on your clinical placements in primary care are the comprehensive electronic patient records on every consulting room desktop. As yet there are few equivalent systems across secondary care in the United Kingdom – though many UK hospital departments have electronic records, hospitals are likely to have a system similar (and integrated with) to that in primary care soon. Many European countries have CIS in all health sectors.

Part of the UK government ambitions include for patient records to be electronic, all referrals to be electronic and also for patients to have access to their own GP records. All this is likely to occur by 2018, before your specialty training jobs are completed. You will need to learn to use these CISs efficiently, safely and accurately – and use them to get the most from the vast capability they have for clinical decision making, audit, research and education. Getting to know the content of these records, how to access data, how to record data so it is useful for others are all key parts of becoming a competent clinician. At best the comprehensive record can support your learning about all aspects of medicine – from the public health aspects including the immunisation record, the social determinants of health perhaps captured in linked family records, to essential information on chronic clinical conditions and their treatment. At worst the sheer scale and complexity of records can be overwhelming, that is why we have included this chapter in the book.

You need to learn, by reading and then doing, what is included in the records and how CISs support excellent patient care. Your primary care placements are an ideal place to get to know and practice and understand these systems. We'll try to guide you in the journey.

Clinical information systems in community practice

In this section we'll try to tell you a little of the background relating to CIS: when they were introduced, why and what functions they offer now. We won't say much about the exact detail, partly because the actual systems change rapidly, and vary across the United Kingdom and other countries. What you need to know are the general principles: what the systems can do, how they can support your learning, how they support clinical practice, how they aid communication – and how all this can go wrong. Many different companies have developed these systems in parallel, with some convergence in recent years. All UK systems operate to a set of common standards with oversight provided by the Health & Social Care Information Centre (HSCIC, 2015).

A further note on learning from different computer systems:

You may find some reluctance to people teaching you skills for a certain type of system. This needs to be challenged. When you do your driving test and lessons you may learn in a Mini, a Polo or a Clio. It doesn't matter which car it is, you learn skills that help you drive any car. You may need to check a few things when you get into a Ferrari – like where are the indicators and how do you switch the lights on. That doesn't mean that you haven't learned, but that you need to indicate at a roundabout or turn your lights on in the dark. These are general principles that you learn, then modify depending on which vehicle you are in. This is the same for CIS – they all have similar capabilities and work according to the same important principles, but each time you use a different one you will need to refine your skills. This chapter will help you learn the important transferrable skills relevant to all systems that you will meet in clinical practice.

Making the most of the CIS in learning and teaching

How is it best to learn about, with and from CIS? We are sure there are many ways, but we'll describe an example of good practice from Leeds Medical School, United Kingdom – developed as a model to share across healthcare providers in one region of the United Kingdom (Yorkshire and the Humber). This approach provides not only a freely

TASK: STARTING OFF YOUR LEARNING

Ask your tutor: If you are not feeling suitably engaged during the consultation, make sure you ask if you can enter data into the CIS. You should have an NHS Smart Card or equivalent access tool to ensure this is done with a clear audit trail and always write 'on behalf of Dr. X' or 'entry confirmed by Dr. Y'. If you haven't got a Smart Card ensure the entry ends 'entered by Joe Student, University of XXX Medical School, on my behalf'*.

But also use this to reflect with your tutors, and discuss information governance processes in the healthcare services in your country.

What to enter?

Consultation records; data from within consultations – blood pressures, alcohol intakes, smoking information; summary of any telephone contacts; information gained from discussions with named patients you see; ideas from home visits. This not only helps you engage in the consultation, but also reinforces what are the important positive and negative findings from the history or examination. A simple concise style suddenly becomes attractive when you have to type it all up!

An example:

'Student entry: myself and a colleague {Fiona Student, UK Medical School} saw this lady at home as part of our learning. She was clearly struggling with opening her jars and turning on the taps and was tearful. She would very much like some advice and support. Discussed with Dr. Tutor who will arrange a follow up with her Rheumatology team. Data entered by Dan Student, UK Medical School'.

available framework for what you might want to learn, but also might provide a useful discussion point with your clinical tutors or medical school. There will be others available too!

Clinical Systems 4 Patient Care (CIS4PC) Project – University of Leeds, UK

http://medhealth.leeds.ac.uk/info/657/cis4pc/

A collaborative project between the Academic Unit of Primary Care and the Yorkshire Centre for Health Informatics has been running at the University of Leeds for the last 5 years, funded via NHS development money. CIS4PC offers a series of reusable learning objects (RLOs) tailored to Tomorrow's Doctors and the MBChB (undergraduate medical degree at Leeds). The teaching uses a live system developed with TPP SystmOne – a web based clinical information system used widely in UK primary care. http://www.tpp-uk.com/products/systmone. Students are able to access the live clinical information system during teaching, enter and retrieve data from prepared patients and learn about clinical information systems and patients at various levels (from essential governance issues, through simple health data, acute illness, consultation skills, chronic illness and prescribing). The work is integrated with students' clinical placements, offering reinforcement of learning across all 5 years of their primary care placements (with NHS Smart Card access enabling applied learning in practice from year 3 onwards).

What do clinical information systems offer in the diagnosis and management of acute illnesses? How do they support your learning of these conditions?

Many patients contact their local GP surgery as they feel acutely unwell (in both professional and lay senses – suddenly unwell and less often very unwell). Depending on the organisation in the practice they may be given advice, seen by a nurse or nurse practitioner or seen by the GP (or perhaps a senior medical student such as you!). Some of these patients will have 'minor' or self-limiting illnesses (coughs, colds etc.) – some the first stages of a more serious acute condition (e.g., sepsis).

Consider and discuss how CIS helps support the nurse or doctor in the diagnosis and treatment of acute illnesses, or in the often fraught differentiation of the presentation of serious early illness from the more mundane majority of viral and self-limiting conditions?

Clinical decision marking/clinical reasoning

Clinical information systems can help diagnosis, differentiation and your own learning in this area. We believe that proficiency in using such diagnostic support is now as essential as being able to use a stethoscope or read an ECG. Diagnosis can occur through algorithms and triage systems as above; but as these systems hold a host of background data on every patient you will see you have to be able to have techniques to quickly and effectively access it.

TASK: USING THE CIS TO GATHER BACKGROUND DATA

First learn by looking: What does your tutor do before he/she sees every patient?

Probably, if they are like us, he/she has a scan of the last few consultations (on-going health issues?); a scan of the major illness summary (heart disease, depression, COPD, cancer?); a look at the repeat medication list. None of these substitutes for a thorough history and a careful listening ear, but 30 seconds gives a vital snapshot on which to base the clinical decision making.

Observe your tutor, and try it for your own patients you see.

What can you learn from the system in 30 seconds?

Practice makes perfect! (Having good systems with updated patient summaries make this all much easier – that is another story!).

What the above doesn't cover, but you may see in some primary care placements (especially out-of-hours or minor illness units), are the use of decision support software embedded within CIS. Many triage systems, increasingly a part of practice as demand increases, offer computer-assisted diagnostic support for nurses or trained non-health professionals. One of the more widely used triage systems that you may be aware of in the United Kingdom at the moment is NHS 111. If you get a chance observe these systems and talk to the staff involved. How does such a system differentiate between a mild allergic rash in a child and a rash due to life threatening meningococcal disease? Are the safeguards built in so cumbersome that they swamp health systems with 'the worried well'?

Clinical management support in primary care

One great challenge in medicine is sharing decisions with patients so they remain empowered and in control of their health. The computer can potentially hinder this (if viewed as a secret repository of information to which the doctor communicates) but at best support it. On a good day we would routinely turn the screen to the patient, share data, graph test results to show them how things are improving or otherwise, look at how risk changes if smoking stops or cholesterol lowering drugs are started and so forth. In acute illnesses many clinicians will share or print patient information leaflets (PALS) or show self-care websites. Many students clinical years are excellent at taking focused histories, but are much less confident at the 'neglected second-half of the consultation' (Elwyn *et al.*, 1999). Discuss that with your tutor, address it and above all practice using the CIS to aid this shared approach to management planning. Start with fairly minor illness such as ear infections, skin problems or similar – using PALS or web-based tools to improve communication in the consultation is an excellent and safe starting point.

Support for learning about 'minor illness'

What we might view as minor self-limiting illnesses, whether coughs, colds, sore throats, sprains, headaches or similar might not appear such to a patient for a wide variety of reasons. This is important and is discussed in Chapter 1.

TASK: MINOR ILLNESSES

Ask your tutor if you can look at his/her last 20 consultations on the systems, and note down the main diagnoses.

What percentage is for 'minor illness'? Why do you think these are 'minor illnesses'? Why would some patients come to the doctor with things others might not?

Discuss you findings and ideas with student colleagues or other learners in the practice or with your tutor.

Remember that previous comments regarding access to records and confidentiality apply!

How do clinical information systems support the management of long-term conditions? How can they support your learning about this vital area of medicine?

So, we hope you have learned a bit about how computers and CISs can help in the diagnosis and treatment of acute and minor illnesses, and helped you start to learn more about this area. But many people think CISs come into their own, and are perhaps essential, in the management of long-term conditions, chronic illnesses – and where there is co-morbidity (two conditions together) or multi-morbidity (several conditions). This is all just as well as 58% of those aged 60 or over are reported to have at least one long-term condition (LTC) with 25% of

these having two or more conditions. https://www.gov.uk/government/
uploads/system/uploads/attachment_data/file/216528/dh_134486.pdf.

You have looked at chronic disease and the United Kingdom's quality
outcome framework (QoF) in Chapter 3. You are aware that there are a
number of conditions where management is closely driven by nationally set targets/guidelines for best practice (and many more where other
national guidance is available for treatment, whichever country you are
studying in). But what does all this mean? How does it work?

Let's think about numbers initially. In the United Kingdom there
are an estimated 300 million general practice consultations a year
(Department of Health, 2008), which is about 90% of all patient contacts
in the NHS (King's Fund: General Practice an overview). All of this
needs to be accurately recorded, stored and made available to access at
any given time. One of the important skills to learn is which part of the
consultation are vital to include (e.g., blood pressure) which parts *may*
be less relevant (recent holiday destination – although of course this may
be vital if the patient presents with diarrhoea or new onset of cough!).
Although all consultations are important to record, some are more vital
than others. Many of these are related to long-term conditions.

Keeping numbers in mind, how do you think any government gets
statistics to release to the public in relation to various illnesses?
Headlines such as 'Highest rate of diabetes record' or 'Greatest rise in
heart disease figures in a decade' come from running reports on data
collected via CISs. This data is only accessible if it is recorded and stored
in a systematic and carefully coded way. This is one of the important
lessons in the management of long-term conditions. Patient records are
only as good as the data that is entered into them – by you!

Let's think about asthma. Every patient who has asthma should have
a number of things checked on an annual basis to ensure their health is
maintained. They need to be seen annually, checked if their symptoms

TASK: GETTING HEALTH STATISTICS FROM PATIENT RECORDS

Ask your GP tutor, practice nurse or practice manager:
• How many patients they have with asthma?
• How many of them have been seen in the last year?
• How many have a recorded peak flow (PEFR)?
• How well does the practice meet its nationally set guidelines for asthma care?

are controlled, diagnosis confirmed and their smoking status recorded and appropriate actions taken following review of their condition.

Reminders, recalls and templates: why is this important to learn?

Studying medicine in primary care provides many opportunities for you as medical students to learn about how to manage a patient's long-term conditions. This is where community placements excel. As GPs we can identify people that do not attend: Are they too ill to attend? Has their illness/condition resolved? Do they not know they should see a clinician annually? This gives information helping us to manage long-terms condition effectively. It supports that part of our work which is population and public health-based and supports individual patients as well. If we did not have CISs we would rely on patients remembering to come in and then on clinicians remembering to check the management of their long-term conditions. This may seem simple, but if you have a patient with COPD, diabetes, thyroid disease who has also recently developed dementia there is a lot to check. It is really useful that there is a little aid memoir or nudge to send you in the right direction, and evidence shows that it works (Roshanov *et al.*, 2013).

In most systems these reminders come in the form of QoF reminders, recalls and templates. Choose a long- term condition and ask your tutor to show you a template and have a look through. Do you think you would be able to do a long-term conditions review with the information included? It may help to think about a condition – why not stay with asthma, read about it (good revision) then imagine the sorts of questions you feel ought to be answered every year to ensure that the patient's condition is treated correctly. Then ask to look at their asthma template. Does it prompt the clinician to answer all your questions? If not discuss them with your tutor.

Templates are part of the systems that can either be standardised or customised by individual practices or users. They help standardise data that is collected by individuals within a practice and they also mean that you need to think less about read codes (see below) when using them as they enter the read codes automatically. These are a good place to look for revision of important topics as most GP practices will have up-to-date information on their templates related to each condition.

Recalls are essentially reminders that can be set up on the system to remind users that things need doing – like a patient's blood test needs completing. But they are better than that, they allow system-wide searches, for example, I could check all 10,500 of my patients to see who was overdue for a blood pressure reading, or who was overdue for a medication review.

Hang on a minute – *Read Codes* – you have lost me!

Read Codes could be compared to a postcode. A postcode consists of many different parts, the first LS may tell you I live in Leeds, the second part (21) may take you to within a few miles of my house, but the entire thing would bring you to my front door (not included). This postcode is decipherable to anyone in the United Kingdom who understands postcodes or any system that understands postcodes – e.g. Google maps. This is the same with a *Read Code*, it takes you to a specific diagnosis like occupational-induced asthma (the entire code). But if you searched for asthma this would still be found in the system. It is a method of labelling diagnoses, symptoms, occupations or actions that can be identified by any system operating this code.

How does the computer identify all those patients with asthma? This is where you come in. If you see a patient in practice that has a new diagnosis – ask your GP tutor how they record it. We hope the answer is 'I code it of course'. Coding is something primary care clinicians should be doing accurately and in a routine way. But it is an essential if is done well! If you learn nothing else from this chapter and your time in practice try to learn two things:

1 How to safely use CISs and patient information – this is a must for Good Medical Practice
2 Learn the importance of codes and the need to accurately use them.

In the early 1980s a GP (Dr. James Read) developed the first diagnostic coding system. The current system is much more refined and goes significantly beyond simply a list of diagnostic codes, but James Read started the whole process. This is not the place to offer details of how this and other coding systems work, but they provide a method of accurately recording information that enables the CIS to function. See: http://systems.hscic.gov.uk/data/uktc/readcodes

If information is not coded the CIS loses its functionality quickly. This is why it is crucial to know about them. Take our asthma patients; if we use free text to write on the computer that a patient has asthma, when you ask the practice manager to tell you how many patients have asthma that person would not be included in the numbers as the systems do not (currently) pick up free text.

TASK

Ask your tutor: You will only learn if you learn actively and get engaged. Have a look, with your tutor's permission, at the last 20 patients they saw: how many had a 'long-term condition?' How did you define and identify that? How many had two or more long-term conditions?

Chose one condition: how many different staff or agencies were involved with that patient's care (and was that clear directly from their entries on the clinical records?) Does the clinical record aid or hinder communication between different parties? How is that communication enhanced? (And have you found the long-term conditions clinic templates yet?)

Learning from clinical guidelines

In Chapter 2 you were introduced to the United Kingdom's long-term condition 'quality and outcomes framework' or 'QoF'. Other countries increasingly have similar frameworks designed to improve quality of the management of long-term conditions across populations. How can these clinical guidelines, including QoF, help you learn? Specifically how can the frameworks and the data linked to them on clinical information systems help you learn?

UK QoF offers an evidence-based framework of the most important conditions, in population terms, in western medicine (and increasingly globally as China, India, Brazil, Russia and many much poorer nations are facing the task of managing diabetes and heart disease; conditions until very recently associated with affluent nations). The information on the appropriate targets for management are available on the CISs, often directly linked to national guidelines (e.g., http://www.nice.org.uk/guidance and http://www.sign.ac.uk/guidelines/index.html in the United Kingdom; and equivalents such as the

KNPG Clinical Guidelines in Holland http://www.kngfrichtlijnen.nl/ index.php/kngf-guidelines-in-english). We suggest you learn from these available guidelines and use them as an aide memoir (or at the very least ensure you are familiar with the conditions included and the principles of management for each).

TASK: DEMENTIA GUIDELINES

Ask your tutor or practice manager to access the national guidance for *dementia* embedded in your CIS.

At best this should include, as it does in the UK QoF, a framework for the diagnosis and recording of a dementia database and guidance on expected standards for diagnosis and care.

Explore similar registers and standards for other conditions currently relevant in your learning and use the data accessed to enhance your knowledge of the illness and its prevalence and management in the placement you are currently attached to.

When you are seeing a patient, have a look first at embedded guidelines/QoF to remind yourself of the management goals and approaches for their key conditions. When you have seen a patient, reflect on the complexities for any given individual of achieving such national guidance (e.g., QoF targets). What gets in the way? Is chasing such targets good medical practice? (Refer Kirkpatrick's work if you want a counter view; Fitzpatrick, 2001.) If you have to do a long-term conditions project or report, use QoF as a framework, or place your patient in the context of a practice summary gained from QoF data (a record usually instantly accessible to the practice manager or clinical governance lead, and remarkably full for most practices: who says financial incentives in medicine don't work?!)

How can clinical information systems support the learning of prescribing (and patient safety)?

As medical students you are often rightly concerned with learning how to prescribe appropriately, effectively and without error. These concerns are justified – prescribing is a key part of medicine and prescribing errors cost lives. One of the great advantages CISs have over manual alternatives is that they introduce 'intelligent prescribing' – that is, built-in guidance to highlight potential dangers in prescribing (excellent for enhancing patient safety) or suggest alternative drugs (often for cost reasons). Equally, the sheer complexity of information provided can itself lead to errors if these systems and their limitations are not fully understood.

Assuming any allergies have been correctly entered on the computer/CIS, at simplest the computer will highlight this where a drug is erroneously prescribed (e.g., Penicillin). Drug interactions are highlighted (e.g., Warfarin and certain antibiotics) as are drug warnings (e.g., need to monitor the full blood count with methotrexate) or advice to pass onto the patient (e.g., avoid alcohol with metronidazole). Senior clinical students will need to know all this information to prepare for clinical practice, but with the huge increase in prescribing complexity you also need to know how to navigate the tools clinicians use to prescribe safely. Multi-morbidity and poly-pharmacy is common in modern medicine and will get ever more complex as new patient-tailored treatments emerge. Most patients with long-term conditions are cared for in the community, it is a great place to learn prescribing skills.

TASK

You will learn by being engaged and active on your clinical placements. In this area we recommend two key activities:

First, do a theoretical exercise; all clinical systems have a dummy patient (usually *Minnie Mouse*, usually with an improbable combination of health problems!). Ask your tutor to demonstrate this. Use it to prescribe some common drugs for common conditions on your modules learning objectives and see what complications you discover. You will find an amazing list of potential prescribing pitfalls and side effects (which as experienced clinicians we accept or actively override through using clinical experience and judgement, but at worst may skim past due to a combination of assumed triviality, time pressures and information overload). Observe your tutor using the system, practice with *Minnie Mouse* or her equivalent, become comfortable with the system and its strengths.

Second, do an exercise with real patients. Ask your tutor if you can help complete consultations. He/she might get as far as recommending the treatment (ideally with your input) but you should ask to 'do the prescription'. Take the hot seat, type the recommended drug in, select the recommended dose. In doing so you'll trigger the lists of interactions, and be posed the awkward choices about alternative formulations or regimes. Again in suggesting this we assume and you should *always* insist on adequate supervision from your tutor.

Third, if you have time ask your tutor to help you choose one of two important drugs relevant to your current learning objectives (e.g., Warfarin and novel anticoagulants for atrial fibrillation). Explore how you would prescribe these for a patient, real if feasible, on the CIS and explore the various safeguards built-in to ensure error is minimised.

Aside from inbuilt features of the CISs, many will have direct online access to other prescribing support, for example, local or national drug formularies; for example, the British National Formulary (www.bnf. org) or national prescribing formulary and guidelines. It is worth ensuring you know how to access such systems, the main advantage being the BNF or equivalent online formulary will be up to date and not an old version left for students as newer ones are obtained by the doctors!

Family medicine, using clinical information systems to learn public health aspects – what do you need to know?

Possibly the most impressive outcomes of CISs, yet one of the least obvious, are their help with the improvement of public health. At medical school public health is one area of medicine that tends to be challenging to learn. It has a central relevance to all of us, yet its comparatively abstract nature means we rarely engage with it on an individual level. Data quality is essential for accurate interpretations of public health. Again the data is only as good as the person who enters it – you.

Consider annual flu outbreaks. Every year countries with temperate climates have a seasonal flu outbreak and every year most developed countries offer vaccination for at risk groups. As a population we vaccinate those at highest risk from the flu (e.g., elderly people; those with long-term conditions such as asthma and diabetes). In 2014 in my practice of 10,500 patients we invited 3295 patients to have their flu jab. These were invited by letter and by text using the information system. These interventions on this scale can only be achieved by computers and codes. But it comes down to your interaction with the system and your coding to enable these lifesaving interventions to take place. We identify and find those at risk from their coded clinical records and invite them to attend for vaccines. This is an annual public health intervention. If you hadn't accurately coded your patient with asthma, then they wouldn't receive a letter inviting them for a vaccine. They could then get the flu and have serious complications that may have been avoided. Clinical information systems are therefore part of the link between individual health and public health. Your ability to code data accurately is a core clinical skill for future practice.

Consider the UK swine flu (H1N1) outbreak in 2009. This was a pandemic (check your epidemiology texts – good revision!). It began as an outbreak, became an epidemic and then a pandemic. Luckily this did not turn out to be as disastrous as predicted yet it still resulted in over 400 deaths in the United Kingdom. Why do we want you to consider this? Public health clinicians take decision based on data, so you may recall the presence of television campaigns, posters and vaccinations being given. These are essential for the health of us as individuals and they also cost the public a lot of money. How do government public health departments decide when to start vaccinating people, offer population-based anti-virals or start asking people to remain at home to isolate an outbreak? This is all based on coding. If a patient is coded as having 'Influenza H1N1' then this feeds into the figures the central bodies see. If the patient is coded as having 'viral upper respiratory tract infection' this patient is not included (even if they actually had H1N1). If data quality is poor from primary care, our reporting figures and public health decision making will be equally poor, with potentially devastating effects.

Let's explore how you embed this knowledge and learn more about public health along the way.

TASK

Imagine the department of health in your country recommends that all those with Rheumatoid arthritis needed flu jabs in future – but not those with low white cell counts. Would the practice you are working in be able to quickly identify all at risk patients?

Test it out:
Ask you tutor or the practice manager to run the relevant searches and consider with them what degree of inaccuracy there may be – and therefore what element of risk if these figures are used for the public health campaigns.

Clinical information systems: supporting learning about communication with patients, and colleagues

We looked briefly in Chapter 4 about how computer systems can either enhance or be detrimental to communication in the consultation. They will be an ever present feature of your life as a clinician – so it is vital you learn to enhance your patient communication with them integrated into your approach. Clinical information systems have a wealth of information you might usefully share with patients or their carers (with permission!). This may range from calculating cardiovascular risks and demonstrating the benefit of smoking cessation or prescribing statins (look it up with your tutor!) or consulting in a balanced patient-centred way, for example, exploring whether or not to undergo genetic testing for breast cancer or do a prostate cancer blood test.

On a more prosaic level you can access and share information on safe prescribing, self-management of back pain or access sites to show pictures of endoscopy, X-ray or scan results. The educational potential is enormous, so is the opportunity to get it wrong (too much information, wrong information, conflicting information etc.). Learning how to best use the system is vital. Your primary care placement is a good time to learn; your tutor will often be skilled at using systems in this way.

TASK

Ask your tutor if you can practice sharing information with one of the patients you see, perhaps within a contained environment such as the long-term conditions clinic when the nurses will often have to communicate risk and risk/benefit decisions relating to lifestyle or prescribing changes.

> Use the tools available to help better communicate risk – you will find a range of options on most systems, linked directly to patient results. Observe how crucial it is for information to be entered correctly (is blood pressure coded, are hospital cholesterol tests available to GP systems, was family history of diabetes of heart disease entered as a free text or coded and available to the risk calculators?).

The authors have little doubt that the use of CISs will increase in future – and you'll see it first in patients' ability to share the screen in the consultation and work with the clinician to formulate diagnosis and treatment plans. Observe your tutor and see how much this already happens. If it doesn't then try it yourself when you have your own consultations with patients – maybe a chance to inform your tutor, or even impress them!

Using clinical information systems in supporting assessment

You may be assessed on your ability to record clinical notes on simple CISs, especially the ability to record data into templates and to follow appropriate Read coding or a similar systematic approach. You can also expect to be assessed about information governance and the professional aspects of good record keeping, confidentiality and data access. It is core to your future clinical practice; misuse is a professional issue just as important as other aspects of professional conduct. For further guidance on these issues refer *GMC Good Medical Practice* (2013). In future we are sure you will have objective structured clinical examination (OSCE) stations which involve you making entry into clinical systems, or retrieve data from them – you heard it here first!

It is likely in future information on the records will be directly useful in your own self-assessment, and after graduation in your continuing professional development (collating automatically everything from prescribing habits to referral patterns or clinical outcome data for your patients). All this will depend on the skills you can use with the systems available. Equally such information will help in assessment of your skills working with clinical teams and for formal workplace-based assessments – allowing authentic assessment on real patients in real time. We suggest you get involved and embrace the technology – not for its own sake or as a gimmick, but to see how it might make your ability to provide excellent, safe and evidence informed patient care in the future.

Clinical information systems: problems and pitfalls

The authors are UK-based GPs and we are justly proud of the fantastic clinical support systems we have on our surgery desktops. High-quality care of patients with multiple and complex health problems would be increasingly unthinkable without them. We are not naïve however – there are problems and pitfalls with all systems, and it is vital you graduate with a healthy scepticism and a critical eye so you can challenge established practice and seek to improve it.

TASK

Ask your tutor, the practice nurses and the administrative staff what they find to be the *problems* of the clinical systems they use – and for those particularly interested read
   Our starter for five to set the conversation going:
   Clinical information systems at worst:

1 Dilute patient confidentiality though widening access to clinical notes – do patients really understand this?

2 Support the promotion of a biomedical model of medicine through emphasising recordable data (blood pressures, cardiovascular risk, etc.) over what often really matters to patients (poor health due to unemployment, abuse, loneliness, poor relationships, depression).

3 Promote a medicine culture – 'a pill for every ill' (perhaps driven by pharmaceutical companies wishing to sell interventions with little limited therapeutic value, for example, look up the quality of evidence for anti-viral drugs or those intended to alleviate the symptoms of dementia).

4 Cause more confusion than they reduce, for example, prescribing support software which highlight every interaction, when in practice only some are significant.

5 Make it almost impossible to get a quick overview of a patient's health problems – there is often simply too much data stored – hard for you as students, hard for doctors pushed for time.

Not only are there potential problems with the systems in their set up and use, but also the systems are intrinsically vulnerable to problems of inappropriate access, data leakage, breaks in confidentiality and other misuse. The same is obviously true of paper records, but the problem magnifies as access becomes easier and attempts are made to make records available to an ever wider range of clinical and administrative staff. Knowing the pitfalls is essential. Let's talk about these and the systems you must insist on to minimise risk.

Smart cards, information governance, confidentiality

Clinical information systems are no different to any other important data system – they need secure access and an ability to record and log who has access to the system, when to leave a clear audit trail in case of error or future challenge. This may seem a little negative or gloomy – but poor entries and poor use of CISs keep the medical defence unions in employment.

Access to CISs in UK primary care settings is via a unique identifier (usually at present a credit card sized NHS Smart Card which doubles as identification badge). In other countries access may be in different ways – but in each case will include a unique identifier and password. The unique identifier protects the patient from unauthorised access to their records, it also protects those accessing records as it details every point of contact, change or transaction with the record so providing a clear audit trail and clinical/administrative path (often useful for complaints or legally).

It is important that as students you similarly have identifiable access; partly to protect you as you make entries, partly to protect doctors and clinicians should any of you be tempted to access data in areas you shouldn't go (if you do so on your login there will be a clear audit trail!)

In many ways Smart Cards or their equivalent for students serve as the dissection room of old, that is, a key moment of transition to becoming clinicians is now being entrusted to access and enter data, and through this becoming part of the clinical team. If you have your Smart Card or equivalent, however limited the access rights, treasure it and take the responsibility you hold seriously.

Obtaining your access to clinical information systems

In the UK medical schools will normally work with their NHS Partners to ensure medical students have access to the NHS data systems, albeit in a very controlled and protected way (with a low level of access compared to qualified staff). The care taken in access reflects abuse in the past, but also human error which will lead to poor quality clinical records if untrained operators have unlimited access. As we suggested above – access, even limited, brings great responsibilities. Other countries will have equivalent ways to provide access and appropriate governance of their clinical systems.

At the time of going to press not all medical schools in the United Kingdom followed this best practice (Jones *et al.*, 2011) and the situation outside the United Kingdom varies widely. The principle of clinical students taking responsibility for material accessed on clinical records is important though. If you are asked to log on to a clinical system for your tutor, you should question this. If you are asked to add data or write up a clinical encounter, it is fine under adequate supervision – but always write something like 'Steven Jones, Yr 4 Medical Student, Newcastle Medical School – supervised by Dr. XXX' as appropriate.

TASK: INFORMATION GOVERNANCE RULES

As a UK-based 'clinical' student, certainly from year 3 onwards, you should have an NHS Smart Card or equivalent to access all CISs you come across and used at all sites. Ask your tutor for more information, read more from the reference section and follow our links to relevant sites.

If you are in a medical school where there is no clear guidance on information governance or no use of NHS Smart Cards, or equivalent safe access to CISs, you may raise this as a concern with the quality officer.

As a clinical student you need safe access to clinical records in order to learn, but have a responsibility to demand that good information governance practice is followed.

Information governance: what do you need to know?

In the United Kingdom there is a clear national guidance on information governance (IG), followed by variable rigour across primary care. It is important you know the principles of this guidance (the detail may change), understand its importance and be prepared to answer questions on it. The underlying principle of IG – and one great benefit of electronic patient records – is that every entry is traceable or 'has an audit trail'. One consequence of this is you should *never* enter data when someone else is logged in (with a possible exception as a student, provided it is clearly labelled – see advice above). See UK Health & Social Care Information Centre for more information http://systems.hscic.gov.uk/infogov.

Keeping information safe is vital – electronic records are comprehensive confidential clinical records, with the benefit of easy accessibility but the potential danger of accidental or intentional revelations of confidential data. Protecting that on a 'need to know' basis is your professional duty as a clinical student, just as it will be your continued responsibility after graduation.

Summary of good practice in IG is as follows:

• Turn off your computer /clinical records when you leave the room (or logout/password protect).
• *Never* leave your Smart card (or equivalent means of access) unattended.
• *Never* lend your Smart card, or ask to borrow a colleague's.
• *Never* share your login/password details.
• Be careful about screen position and visibility if a third party is in a consultation (even if a close relative such as husband, wife or parent of any child above the age of 14).

TASK

If you are in UK general practice* ask your tutor who is the 'Caldecott Guardian' and ask him/her explain what the role entails and what responsibilities it brings. See what the practice policies are on IT governance. How do these policies improve data security and how do they hinder communication? Discuss this with peers and your tutor(s).

*In other countries responsible officers for IG will also be there – similarly explore their roles.

Clinical information systems: projects, audit and research

Some of you may be really interested in computers, data and information systems. Some of you may recognise how important they are or feel challenged by needing to know all this stuff. Getting more immersed in the subject through a special project or student selected component of work may be for you. Helping practice staff run an audit or do a small research study using the information systems will not only help you learn, but may also get you a poster, prize or publication.

TASK

Share any project ideas you have with your placement or personal tutor or someone appropriate from the medical school. Look carefully at the guidance and scale of the project you need to do to complete your assessment. Think about questions best answered by use of the CISs. This could be a wide range of things: how they are actively used in the consultation to help share information with patients (a research question); how many patients on statins have their liver function tests monitored regularly (audit); how the quality of data summary in the over 75s may be improved in the practice (project work). Choose something that will help you improve your skills as well as help the practice answer a worthwhile question.

Remember you are now part of the team, you stopped being 'just a student' at the end of *Freshers' week*. This is medicine; we are all trying to improve patients' lives.

Summary

One of the great strengths of primary care is the quality of its CISs, essential to support the ever more complex patients and families we look after. Your community placements are ideal as a base to learn the rules and skills of good CISs – skills which will be essential in both primary and secondary care when you graduate. We have shared tips about how to find out more about these systems, but have also explored how they can enhance you learning of clinical medicine – both acute and relating to long-term conditions and complex multi-morbidity. Finally we have suggested some ideas to really enhance your understanding and competence in the various tools these systems have – including the ability to search for data, link individual and population health and conduct audit of clinical quality.

References

Department of Health Departmental Report (2008) The Health and Personal Services Programmes TSO (The Stationary Office) Norwich, UK. Available at: http://webarchive.nationalarchives.gov.uk/20130107105354/http://www.dh.gov.uk/prod_consum_dh/groups/dh_digitalassets/@dh/@en/documents/digitalasset/dh_084910.pdf (accessed 24 March 2009).

Elwyn G, Edwards A, Kinnersley P (1999) Shared decision-making in primary care: the neglected second half of the consultation. The British Journal of General Practice 49(443):477–482.

Fitzpatrick M (2001) The Tyranny of Health: Doctors and the Regulation of Lifestyle. London: Routledge.

GMC (2009) Tomorrow's Doctors. http://www.gmc-uk.org/Tomorrow_s_Doctors_1214.pdf_48905759.pdf (accessed 15 July 2015).

GMC (2013) Good Medical Practice. http://www.gmc-uk.org/static/documents/content/Good_medical_practice_-_English_0914.pdf (accessed 22 March 2015).

HSCIC (2015) Health & Social Care Information Centre. http://systems.hscic.gov.uk/gpsoc (accessed 22 March 2015).

Jones RG, Mehta MM, McKinley RK (2011) Medical student access to electronic medical records in UK primary care. Education for Primary Care 22(1):4–6.

Roshanov PS, Fernandes N, Wilczynski JM, Hemens BJ, You JJ, Handler SM, et al. (2013) Features of effective computerised clinical decision support systems: meta-regression of 162 randomised trials. BMJ 346:f657.

Select Committee for Health (2007) http://www.publications.parliament.uk/pa/cm200607/cmselect/cmhealth/422/42207.htm (accessed 7 July 2015).

Chapter 8 **Supporting learning in primary care using social media and other technologies**

With Jonathon Tomlinson

Chapter 8 looks at the use of social media in medical education, and particularly where this and other use of technology in learning may contribute to your learning on placement. It is intended to help those of you with no knowledge at all and those with a little knowledge who would like to know more. Share it with your tutors also, they may be interested or get inspired!

The chapter includes links and references to material for further reading. Some of the initial excitement and concern about social media in higher education has passed. As the dust settles we believe that the best institutions and educators will be encouraging its use to your advantage. Community placements are often a place for innovation, and we encourage you to both learn and where needed educate your tutors in this field.

This chapter has been written by GPs who have extensive experience of teaching undergraduate medical students in community and general practice settings across a variety of settings. We offer our insight from this perspective.

By the end of this chapter you should be able to:

- understand the basic principles of digital and information literacy
- appreciate what is a digital profile and what is meant by digital professionalism
- start to use, or find new ways to use, social media within your medical education and specifically on your community placements
- learn about how patients are using social media to contribute to medical education

---

How to Succeed on Primary Care and Community Placements, First Edition.
David Pearson and Sandra Nicholson.
© 2016 John Wiley & Sons, Ltd. Published 2016 by John Wiley & Sons, Ltd.

What we are not covering in this chapter is the extensive range of online learning, virtual learning and e-learning that will be increasingly core to your education in most medical schools. We are taking this as read, hopefully correctly. We do have concerns that good community-based learning must be supported by excellent online learning and easy access for both tutor, practice and students to the University/medical schools systems – if this is not the case you should certainly raise the problems with you tutor or faculty. The primary care/community learning environment must be as well connected as other NHS/hospital sites – and probably more so given your potential increased isolation when on smaller placements.

Social media in your primary care placements

Ever increasing numbers of students, doctors, medical educators, professional organisations and patients are sharing educational resources online. Medical journals are now all available online and many, like the *British Medical Journal* and *the New England Journal of Medicine* have specially formatted versions for reading on mobile devices. Medical schools like Leicester in the United Kingdom and Harvard in the United States are uploading educational videos to YouTube that can be watched by anyone, anywhere at any time. Healthcare professionals and medical students are writing blogs and using Facebook, Twitter and other sites to organise medical education. Conferences that involve time, travel and high registration fees are being shared for free by video and audio, blogs and twitter. Medical education is not bound by the geographical or temporal confines of medical school any more. We all need to keep up to date with medical research, ethics and policy using online resources which increasingly include social media, so we also need to learn the skills to be sceptical, connected and collaborative online. You will often have the time to explore these aspects of supported medical education while on your primary care placements, you may find your tutor is an 'early adopter' of new ideas and as you are more isolated physically from your University or clinical base you'll benefit from using social, medical and online learning resources all the more.

> **TASK**
>
> - Which online journals can you access from your community placement? Which ones does your tutor access? Which ones are most effective online and why?
> - Search YouTube for medical education tutorials. Discuss with your tutor: Can you find anything from a patient perspective? How can you be sure of quality of information? What role should they have in supporting your learning?
> - Look at Health talk online http://healthtalkonline.org/ for a wide range of videos by patients talking about their experience of illness. Discuss them with colleagues.

When media becomes social media

Media becomes social when there is dialogue and interaction. Just as a traditional lecture is enhanced by questions and discussion, social media thrives because of feedback and debate. One example you might be familiar with are the 'rapid responses' in the *British Medical Journal*. They allow readers, including medical students and patients, to debate articles published online with the authors and other readers. The ex-editor of *BMJ*, Richard Smith, is so enthusiastic about this post-publication peer-review that he has advocated scrapping pre-publication peer review (Smith, 2011a, b). Comments from all over the world involving professors, patients, specialists and students flatten traditional hierarchies, for example, a *BMJ* article about the use of Wikipedia citations attracted comments from several professors, but it was a medical student who attracted most votes for explaining that it is possible to give a time-specific citation (McKechnie, 2014). The wonderful thing about social media is the opportunity to share a very wide range of perspectives on different problems and to share the best and most interesting medical education resources in the world very quickly. Once you are comfortable using social media for medical education you can quickly find answers to all sorts of questions.

You will find that your community placement tutors are often innovators or early adopters of new ideas and technology. You will often have a longer more intimate relationship with tutors in primary or community care than in other aspects of your medical education – use this time to explore innovation using social or online media – and use the expertise and enthusiasm of tutors you meet who are passionate and active in this field.

TASK

- Find an interesting article from the latest edition of BMJ or student BMJ or an equivalent clinical medical journal. Read the 'rapid responses' online. Who is contributing and what is the added value?
- Look at the new BMJ series, 'What Your Patient is Thinking' and read some of the responses.
- Discuss this with your peers on placement and/or your tutor. Is there anything you could contribute? How could this support your future learning?

Social media landscape

Any online media, from *BMJ* to Amazon, Facebook to Wikipedia, which allows users to contribute, is 'social media'. Most Internet activity is user-generated with Facebook and Twitter having over a billion users each and sites like YouTube for videos, Flickr for photographs, Blogs for mixed media, Slideshare and Prezi for presentations and so on. All of these sites have useful material for medical education. It is authored, critiqued and re-configured by users including academicians, clinicians and medical students. You can use social bookmarks, web feeds and tags to share, save and organise material; for an example, see: http://brainandbehaviour.wikispaces.com/?responseToken=0620ef42e25457 b515e05863acd51a431

One of the benefits of community placements, sometimes seen as a drawback, is frequently free time in the middle of the day. This is a time that could be earmarked particularly to engage with social media in this context, and discuss the pros and cons with your peers (both virtually and those with you on placement).

TASK

- Look at one of the sites listed above that you are less familiar with and read some of the comments.
- Can you find examples of shared learning relevant to your development as a doctor? How might you best access such learning?

- Think about how you share online information with your friends? Which ways are most effective?
- How could you use this for medical education?

Your online profile and digital professionalism

As you go through your medical student training you are not only learning how to be a doctor, but you are also becoming a professional. High standards of professional behaviour are expected while you are a medical student, especially in later clinical years. This means you need to be very aware/mindful of your online profile and 'digital footprint' a record of your activity online) – make sure it supports this expected level of professional behaviour. You may also wish to develop a specific online profile. This usually includes a photograph, your name and a brief biography.

TASK

- Try searching online for a role model, perhaps your GP tutor online or course lead, to see what information is available, how they conduct themselves and what impressions peers, employers or patients might make of them.
- Ask a friend to Google you and do the same to your profile. What impression do you think patients and tutors will have if they look you up online?
- Look at the GMC and the Royal College of GPs guidelines for digital professionalism, covering the use of profiles and behaviour online. Be aware that there are different levels of privacy and that some experts are warning that it is becoming harder to separate personal and professional identities online.

Your digital footprint

The contributions you make online are your 'digital footprint'. Like your profile, you should consider it searchable and therefore public and permanent. Many doctors and students are put off by social media because of this.

Before I started using social media I wrote for Inside Time, the national prisoners' newspaper. It is freely available inside every prison in the UK and I answered about a dozen letters a month. I had to provide a photograph of myself and a brief biography which was printed in the paper. Initially I was worried about this, in case a prisoner was offended by my advice and came looking for me, but I was assured that all of the Inside Time contributors did the same thing and they had never had any problems. I wrote for the paper for about 3–4 years without any negative repercussions. My attitude to social media was that if it was OK to share my professional profile with the nation's prisoners, it was probably safe to share it online. My profile on twitter includes my full name and a brief biography with a link to more information:@mellojonny East London GP, NIHR research fellow - medical education, ethics and professional behaviour. Patient advocate. Policy critic Hackney, London. https://abetternhs. wordpress.com/

(Jonathon)

Although many social media sites including Facebook allow private conversations, none of them should be considered completely safe and confidential. Patient details should *never* be revealed.

Doctors and patients online

This section highlights what you can do and how you can learn from engaging with social media while on your community placements.

TASK

- Find out if your practice uses social media?
- How does it contribute to patient care?
- Does it just broadcast or is there interaction with their patients?

Many doctors and medical students worry about patients contacting them online via social media but in my experience this rarely happens and is usually easily and politely dealt with. The public are fascinated with the lives of medical professionals, including medical students and you will be judged on your tact, courtesy, kindness, professionalism, wit and wisdom. Because of this, social media can help to nurture this kind of behaviour and can help to teach us behave like professionals.

Mark Brown; @Markoneinfour wrote the following on Twitter about patients and professionals interacting on social media:

Social media is in some ways the latest village square or local cafe. It's a place where people check in to hear the latest news, catch up with friends, debate, flirt, ferment revolution and/or swap dirty jokes. In short, it's a place where people do people stuff. Social media is where people are.

https://shirleyayres.wordpress.com/2014/03/04/guest-post-markoneinfour-social-media-and-public-professionals-expo14nhs/

There are a lot of patients, including Mark, who use social media to write about their experience of illness and are very keen to share these with doctors and medical students. For the most part, they want to help us learn more.

TASK

Have a look at blogs relevant to your learning (e.g., pain, cancer, mental health or diabetes – any area you focus on due to shared experiences or directly linked to your current learning objectives). Examples include:
Chronic pain: http://noonegetsflowersforchronicpain.wordpress.com/ or
Cancer: http://drkategranger.wordpress.com/
Schizophrenia: https://sectioneduk.wordpress.com/
Bipolar: https://purplepersuasion.wordpress.com/
Diabetes: http://ninjabetic1.blogspot.co.uk/
- What are the differences between what patients write online and what they say when you are with them?
- How does learning from these blogs enhance other learning?
- How does it help reinforce face-to-face learning from patients?
- What do these add to a medical history?
- What extra insight can be gleaned?

Digital literacy and information literacy

Digital literacy refers to the skills required to operate digital technology. *Information literacy* is the ability to find and manage information online. As tutors we sometimes assume that as students you know more about social media and understand digital technology because you are 'digital natives'. That isn't always however the case. An excellent paper about information literacy suggests that although many students conduct a lot of their social life online this is not the same as being digitally literate or information literate (Bhimani, 2011). Paperless medical student Joshua James Harding is an exception: he has written a valuable guide to what is possible (Harding, 2013), but there is an enormous range of ability among both students and teachers and we can learn from each other.

Advantages of using digital devices used with apps like *Evernote* or *Noteability* to organise notes include:

- Linking notes to other material such as textbooks, journal articles, websites, videos etc.
- Having access to your notes wherever you are
- Being able to easily edit your notes with new material
- Not losing your notes
- Sharing material with other students and teachers

Not all placement tutors welcome students bringing mobile devices to teaching sessions, perhaps because they assume that students are not paying attention or that they are playing games or organising their social life online. Equally, many tutors and indeed patients will be anxious about you looking at your phone or tablet in the consultation if they don't know what you are doing. Explain what you are doing so that your tutor and/or patients don't suspect you of not paying attention, or ask permission to use a phone or tablet ('I am just double checking the appropriate dose of your new prostate drug on the Internet' or 'The national clinical guidance on this suggests we re-check your blood test in 3 months') and show them what you are doing. You might be able to teach them something too.

When you are in independent clinical practice it is inconceivable that technology and information sharing won't be more a part of every consultation in primary care – you can help move this new form of working forward through dialogue with your tutor and sharing ideas.

Primary care and community placements are often a good place to develop these essential skills of *information literacy*. First, students on such placements will often have project work to do, and be accessing online supportive material, so you are practicing the skills. Second, you will often have strong support from your tutor/mentor – and the space and time to debate what's a good source of information and what's not as good a source. Use the expertise if it exists to discuss information literacy – the checklist below may be of benefit if your tutor is also unsure.

Brabazon (2012) lists ten points for consideration which forms a useful reminder: http://www.uta.edu/huma/agger/fastcapitalism/9_1/brabazon9_1.html

1 Who authored the information?
2 What expertise does the writer have to comment?
3 What evidence is being deployed here?
4 What genre is the document? Journalism, academic paper, blog, polemic?
5 Are the site/document/reports funded by an institution?
6 What argument is being made?
7 When was the text produced?
8 Why did this information emerge at this point in history?
9 Who is the audience?
10 What is not being talked about?

When assessing a piece of student work, the marker will often start with their references which can reveal a lot about their information literacy.

Social media sites: Facebook, Twitter, Blogs, Wikis, YouTube, Slideshare/Prezi, Scoop.it/Pinterest

This is a book about learning medicine in primary care, not about learning how to use social media. However we argue the boundary is increasingly blurred – and being literate and active in different social media domains is essential for your learning – and to help better engage with both patients and your colleagues in medicine. The following section is a very brief description of some social media sites. For more comprehensive information, please see the references at the end. There are thousands to choose from, which can give the impression that it is impossible to keep up, or that anything written in a book will be out of date by the time of publication, so we have highlighted those that have shown greatest popularity and resilience rather than the very latest.

If you are engaging with any or all of these sites please be *extremely careful* to follow any regulations set by your own medical school. Do not risk getting into hot water about disclosure, confidentiality or other issues of professionalism – if in any doubt don't post something and ask first.

Facebook

Facebook was originally developed for college and university students and now has well over a billion users. It heads the list of social media sites simply because it is where almost all medical students conduct their lives online. There are advantages of bringing education to where students are congregating and making use of technology they are familiar with, but what goes on here, even among university students is more akin to hanging out rather than creative learning. The theory of social learning (Bandura, 1963) would suggest that as humans we learn through meaningful social encounters – and inevitably when such encounters are with fellow students or medical peers, part of the outcome will be enhanced medical education. Whether this is a positive or negative learning experience depends, as with face-face encounters, on the groups you interact with (with much evidence of the disadvantage of social learning with disruptive colleagues as well as the positive influence of strong learning groups).

TASK

Discuss with your faculty or tutor the possibility of setting up a Facebook page, Wikispaces or WhatsApp to support learning through your community placement. Be mindful of any medical school rules before you proceed.

Help the less confident members of the group, including your tutor(s) if necessary, to use it.

Think about what material will be on it, what privacy levels you need and how alerts will be set up.

Discuss with your tutor(s) or faculty the educational benefits of such a group and try to evaluate at the end of placement whether some or all of these have been met.

Blogs

Blog is short for 'web log', literally an online diary. Some patient blogs are discussed before.

I have been writing a blog; https://abetternhs.wordpress.com since 2009. They can be used to present work or research or reflective writing. I have published essays about subjects like 'how doctors respond to patients with chronic pain', 'how lonely patients present to doctors' and 'empathy and medical education'. Readers can make comments which might include their own experiences, corrections or suggestions for further reading. They have enabled me to challenge health policy, promote general practice and explore the relationships between doctors and patients. I get feedback from policy makers, GPs, patients and medical students, much of it very supportive.

(Jonathon Tomlinson)

There are some excellent blogs by medical students, such as http://crazylifemedstudent.blogspot.co.uk/ with advice for other students about interviews and survival on the wards.

There are also blogs about medical education by Natalie Lafferty at: http://mededelearning.wordpress.com/ and Anne Marie Cunningham at: http://wishfulthinkinginmedicaleducation.blogspot.co.uk/

Blogging doctors include:

Dr. Laura Jane, a respiratory doctor: http://drlj.me/

Dr. Partha Kaur is a consultant diabetologist: http://nhssugardoc.blogspot.co.uk/

TASK

- Read some blogs from medical students and professionals. What useful insights do you get from them and how do you think they provide communities of learning and peer support?
- Read some blogs from primary care nurses, general practitioners/family doctors or community health specialists. How are these sites used to support good clinical practice or service improvement or even highlight areas of concern?
- Find an interesting blog and subscribe to updates using an RSS feed.

Twitter

Why is *Twitter* important to you as medical students? What is its value in medical education and on community placements? We have two main reasons for including it: first, very many leaders and shapers in primary care and general practice have active Twitter accounts – and you might find following them to be a great way to get a real feel of the organisation, strengths, weaknesses and tensions of medicine in this less familiar arena.

There are certain times of the week when people with particular interests join in together to discuss a subject that is labelled with a #, for example, #meded for medical education or #mhchat for mental health chat, #ecgclass or #twitjc for Twitter Journal club. #twitjc also has its own website: http://www.twitjc.com/. People joining the discussions have included the author(s) of the paper being discussed, academics, patients, other health professionals, medical and nursing students and so on. Anyone can contribute or simply read the tweets. Search for the tweets using '#twitjc' or save interesting tweets by clicking the 'Favourite' star. It is a great forum to share different perspectives and expertise. There are several beginners' guides that can help, but like all types of social media, prepare your profile, watch how others conduct themselves and joining in a conversation is the best way to learn.

TASK

One of the strengths of primary care placements is to learn mental health and how mental health is intimately linked to physical and social health.

To appreciate different perspectives on mental health during your community placement, search Twitter for #MHChat or #meded or patients like @BipolarBlogger or @Sectioned Find out who is contributing and read some of the comments and links they share. Think about the value of this interdisciplinary discussion in relation to your learning objectives for the year or module you are currently doing. If in doubt about how to align this with your learning objectives please discuss this with your tutor. He/she will be delighted to try to focus and facilitate your learning

Wikispaces

Wikispaces is a kind of simple blog that can be used to share information online and edited by any number of users. It is something your tutor may use to share information and resources (alongside and hopefully complimentary to the medical School's virtual learning environment [VLE]). Equally you may wish to explore their use in sharing information with your peers.

Instead of hand-outs and emails, as students you can check the *Wikispaces* where the timetable and reading material is available. Explore the potential of using *Wikispaces* with your tutor.

An example from Jonathon's own teaching is shown in Figure 8.1.

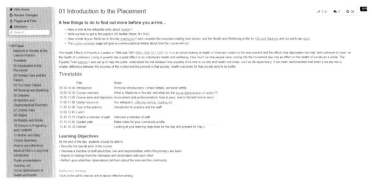

Figure 8.1 Using *wikispace* to help support placements

YouTube

YouTube is the second most popular search engine after Google and has more than a billion user visits a month. Users can watch/upload/recommend/share and comment on videos. Many medical schools, including Harvard, have their own YouTube channels with medical education videos online that students from any university can watch anywhere at any time (Harvard Medical School, 2014). Hundreds of other organisations and individuals have uploaded excellent quality medical education videos, but like any online material, you will need the information literacy to be able to rate its quality and arguably a sceptic mind. If in doubt use your tutor to discuss sites and content.

Let's look at an example of relevance to primary care. The US Mayo Clinic has over 1000 videos online. The author has used their representation of a 'scintillating scotoma' to teach medical students and reassure patients with migraines (Mayo Clinic, 2014). 'Scintillating scotomas' are hard for patients to describe and they have appreciated it and felt reassured when they realise that other patients suffer the same symptoms. In less than 5 minutes it is possible to watch the video and read a significant number of comments and have a very good understanding about different visual auras. The value of social media is in the comments left by patients about their own experience. Look up this and other examples, use them to reinforce learning of common problems you see in primary care, discuss the use of YouTube material with you tutor and practice enhancing your information sharing with patients using such resources.

TASK: USING YOUTUBE ON YOUR PLACEMENTS

Find *YouTube* videos for one of the conditions you are meant to be currently covering on your curriculum, for example, cardiovascular or respiratory examinations.
- Which ones do you think are best and why?
- Explore how you might bookmark them and share them with your colleagues (or tutors).

Find YouTube videos made by patients which link to a condition you have seen with your primary care tutor. Which ones are most effective from an educational perspective?
- Do they help enhance your learning, and why?
- Share your ideas with your colleagues and tutor.

Scoop.it/Pinterest

Scoop.it and *Pinterest* allow users to collate and present material on a virtual pinboard. *Pinterest* seems to be a favoured site for wedding planning and interior decoration, whereas *Scoop.it* has more academic/educational material, but there is useful material on both sites. As students in primary care you might explore both sites and discuss contents with your colleagues or tutor. For example you could use images about public health and obesity to support your learning about the use of shame and stigma in public health campaigns, for example, those compiled by Australian sociologist Deborah Lupton (Lupton, 2015).

Summary

Learning medicine in the community setting takes you into a dispersed learning environment, potentially isolated from colleagues and central medical school facilities. Of all your places of learning it is essential you are able to access and use virtual learning and social media sites to maximise opportunity to learn and enhance the essential interaction with patients, staff and your tutor.

Familiarise yourself thoroughly with your school's virtual learning environment and use it on placement. Make sure your tutor(s) engages and interact with it. You can support this and point out where the essential information on the curriculum is held.

Explore and use a variety of social media forms to enhance learning – share ideas with colleagues. There are many, many more social media sites not mentioned here that may prove to be more useful, more popular and more enduring than the ones we have highlighted. Social media in a multitude of guises is here to stay – as students join in, get involved and help enhance not only your learning, but also your ability to share information and communicate with patients. Remember in doing so you need to be extremely mindful to comply with your medical schools' policies – and very mindful to avoid breaches of professional behaviour, especially confidentiality.

References

Bandura, A. (1963) Social Learning and Personality Development. New York: Holt, Rinehart, and Winston.

Bhimani, N. (2011) Information literacy: a 21st century graduate skill. Middlesex Journal of Education Technology 1 (1), 1–7.

Brabazon, T. (2012) Time for a digital detox? First Capitalism 9 (1). Available from http://www.uta.edu/huma/agger/fastcapitalism/9_1/brabazon9_1.html (accessed 12 March 2015).

Brown, M. (2014) Social media and public professionals. https://shirleyayres.wordpress.com/2014/03/04/guest-post-markoneinfour-social-media-and-public-professionals-expo14nhs/ (accessed 12 March 2015).

Harding, J.J. (2013) Being a paperless medic. Insights 26 (3). http://uksg.metapress.com/content/t1536635x83n7274/fulltext.pdf (accessed 12 March 2015).

Lupton, D. (2015) Fat Culture. Pinterest: http://www.pinterest.com/dalupton/fat-culture/ (accessed 7 July 2015).

Mayo Clinic. (2014) Migraine Visual Aura. YouTube: http://youtu.be/qVFIcF9lyk8 (accessed 12 March 2015).

McKechnie, D. (2014) Re: References that anyone can edit: review of Wikipedia citations in peer reviewed health science literature. BMJ. http://www.bmj.com/content/348/bmj.g1585/rr/689515 (accessed 12 March 2015).

Smith, R. (2011a) Twitter to replace peer-review? BMJ Blogs. http://blogs.bmj.com/bmj/2011/01/26/richard-smith-twitter-to-replace-peer-review/ (accessed 24 March 2014).

Smith, R. (2011b) What is post-publication peer review? BMJ Blogs. http://blogs.bmj.com/bmj/2011/04/06/richard-smith-what-is-post-publication-peer-review/ (accessed 12 March 2015).

Further resources

Clinical Examinations. Leicester University. http://www.youtube.com/playlist?list=PLC4EEBF6359D030E0 (accessed 12 March 2015).

Creative Commons: About the Licenses. https://creativecommons.org/licenses/ (accessed 12 March 2015).

Evernote. http://Evernote.com (accessed 15 July 2015).

Ffolliet. Guns don't kill, bullet points do. Slideshare http://www.slideshare.net/ffolliet/guns-dont-kill-bulletpoints-do# (accessed 12 March 2015).

Harvard Medical School (2014) YouTube. https://www.youtube.com/user/harvardmedicalschool (accessed 12 March 2015).

Notability. http://www.gingerlabs.com (accessed 15 July 2015).

Social bookmarking (Wikipedia). http://en.wikipedia.org/wiki/Social_bookmarking (accessed 12 March 2015).

Social Media Highway Code. Royal College of General Practitioners. http://www.rcgp.org.uk/social-media (accessed 12 March 2015).

Tags. Wikipedia. http://en.wikipedia.org/wiki/Tag_(metadata) (accessed 12 March 2015).

Web Feed. Wikipedia. http://en.wikipedia.org/wiki/Web_feed (accessed 12 March 2015).

Chapter 9 **Assessment, feedback and quality assurance**

With Mark Williamson

Assessment drives learning, so this is important!

We hope to do three things in this chapter. First, help you to understand what is the nature of assessment in your primary care placement and how to get the most from it; second, help you get the most useful and constructive feedback you can and third, to look at your role in improving the quality of your placements and teaching for those who will come after you.

Assessment includes all the elements by which you, and your tutors, can judge your progress against the set course objectives in both primary care and medicine in the widest sense. We include in that formal assessment, self-assessment, peer assessment and formative assessments as set by the tutor or School. Assessment drives learning, so this chapter should be as important to you as it is to your tutors. We hope to help you understand what the elements of assessment are likely to be in your primary care placement, how to succeed in these assessments and how in doing so you get the most from the placement.

Feedback is also a vital part of your student journey. We want to help you know what to expect from feedback in primary care, help you get the most useful and constructive feedback you can from tutors, the primary health team and patients – and how we can encourage you to give high quality feedback to your peers, your tutors and the School.

How to Succeed on Primary Care and Community Placements, First Edition.
David Pearson and Sandra Nicholson.
© 2016 John Wiley & Sons, Ltd. Published 2016 by John Wiley & Sons, Ltd.

Quality assurance is important to you as future doctors. As students you have a vital role both in relation to teaching quality and to clinical quality. Most students welcome the chance to help modify or improve the quality of clinical educational placements for those who will come after them. However, you may have thought less about how your role as students helps improve the patient experience, but this was one area raised recently in the United Kingdom by the *Francis report* into poor standards of care in the Mid. Staffordshire hospitals (Francis Report, 2013).

By the end of this chapter you should be able to:

- understand the nature and likely process of assessment on primary care placements.
- get more ideas for receiving and disseminating feedback to better help your development into a rounded health professional.
- understand how as a student you can contribute fully to quality assurance processes, and what extra you can do if you are particularly interested in this area.

Assessment in your primary care placement

Principles of assessment

This section is about the principles which underpin the assessment process in learning within primary care placements. It looks at some important issues which may affect your chances of success in achieving your goals.

One of the great potential strengths of primary care placements is their ability to allow authentic assessment. In general you get more continuity of tutors in primary care, you are better known, you are with a tutor for longer periods and are more visible. (There are obvious exceptions to this, and obvious good practice in hospitals – but we believe the general point is valid and will chime with your own experience.) For all these reasons tutors should be able to offer very accurate assessments of your performance – both formative and summative. What is more they should be in a very good position to assess both your directly observed clinical and communication skills and your skills at interacting with colleagues, staff and patients, that is, your team-working skills, inter-professional skills and professionalism. Use these opportunities.

Types of assessment

Formative assessment is that which won't contribute directly to your progression, grades or awards. However it is no less important for that. Indeed, formative assessment is critical to the effectiveness of the educational process. At best it guides you about progress, offers an honest status report of where strengths and weaknesses lie, and frequently tutors feel able to be blunter and more specific than in summative tests.

Summative assessment by contrast counts directly. It will affect your progress. It has to be reliable and valid but it also has to be useful – multiple choice tests won't tell you how well you work with colleagues or patients – directly observed workplace-based assessment is best for that.

Much of your assessment on primary care placements will come from your tutor(s). Ideally, however, there will be opportunities for *peer assessment* (your colleagues being encouraged to rate you and give feedback), from *multisource assessment* (contribution for practice staff, nurses, those with on placements), from direct patient assessment (perhaps with multisource feedback – but frequently as formative if your tutor encourages it).

Finally, *self-assessment* is what it says 'on the tin' – using resources online or written to assess against benchmarks and reflect in order to improve. Your tutor should encourage this – ideally linked to key areas of your learning relevant to the current placements. Use these opportunities.

Assessments in medical courses, what should you expect?

TASK: ENGAGE WITH YOUR TUTOR

Suggest your tutor looks at your learning plan and your record of previous assessments, even if you are not proud of it or don't agree with it all. You are on placement to learn. You need to ensure your tutor has all the tools and information with which to help you.

Make sure your tutor is aware of your prior learning, the stage of the course, the schools placement objectives and of course your assessment needs. Make sure that it is very clear early in the placement.

If the tutor seems unsure, gently give the information, or where needed direct them to the medical school website/virtual learning environment (VLE).

It is your education, engage and make your tutor's job easier!

UK medical schools are regulated externally, by the QAA and the GMC, and internally assessed against the quality systems and processes defined by those organisations (or their equivalents in countries outside the United Kingdom). Other nations will have equivalent governance bodies – but this serves as a useful example. The UK Quality Code for Higher Education is developed and maintained by the Quality Assurance Agency for Higher Education (QAA).[1] The important element of this code for student assessments is the concept of threshold standards and academic quality. The former are the minimal level of achievement that you have to reach on your program of study in medical education, and these should not vary from one higher education provider to another. The latter is how well your school delivers teaching, supports your education with staff and resources, and how you are assessed. This section will help you understand what the school is expected to deliver to support you in your learning.

Tomorrow's Doctors (GMC, 2009a) is a document referenced throughout this book and is essential reading at least for UK medical students. We have picked out a few key points from the GMC's linked guidance on assessment (GMC, 2009b) and looked to see how these are relevant to you on a primary care placement (the principles will be equally important for those of you outside the United Kingdom):

- GMC TD (2009b) Supplementary Guidance on Assessment Para 19: *Medical schools should take an overarching strategic and systematic approach to assessment that fits with the rest of the curriculum.* Therefore, your assessments should relate to the published learning outcomes for the primary care placements, which must in turn relate directly to those of the GMC's Tomorrow's Doctors. You will get the most out of the placements, and do best in your assessments, if you understand how the curriculum is designed and operates at your medical school and in your primary care placements. Explore this with your tutor.
- GMC TD (2009b) Supplementary Guidance on Assessment Para 32: *In developing and reviewing assessment methods, medical schools should consider validity, reliability, generalisability, feasibility, fairness,*

---

[1] http://www.qaa.ac.uk/en

educational impact, cost-effectiveness, acceptability and defensibility. These criteria will shape how the school's assessments are designed. If you consider the primary care placement's assessments are not valid, fair or reliable, then discuss with your student representatives who can discuss any concerns with the responsible members of faculty. Assessment bias from individual tutors is always a concern for students and the faculty; equally professional judgement will always be the central element of any work place based assessment in a profession. Using multiple sources of opinion within assessment usually ensures your assessment will be valid and fair, but you should always feel empowered to question surprises.

- GMC TD (2009b) Supplementary Guidance on Assessment Para 60: *Medical schools should provide clear, accessible and timely information to students and staff.* With regards to your primary care placements you should expect:
  - ○ Clear information on the objectives for your primary care placements, and how achieving these will be assessed (accepting these are often integrated with other learning in other clinical settings).
  - ○ Clear information on the nature and expected standards within assessments.
  - ○ Good formative assessment and appropriate feedback early in placements to guide your progress (summative exam results should never be a surprise).
  - ○ Clarity about the nature of feedback you can expect after assessments and at the end of your placement.

What types of assessment should you expect on your primary care placements?

Assessment of contribution

All medical schools will expect explicit standards of attendance, behaviour, dressing and contribution to the educational experience for yourself and your colleagues. These are essential elements of becoming a professional. These factors are rigorously observed in primary care, sometimes more so than other areas of the curriculum as you are likely to be a highly visible member of a small team for longer than in many secondary care placements.

Assessments based on professional judgement are an important element of primary care placements and will start as soon as you make contact with your placement provider or tutor. The importance of behaving appropriately from the outset is therefore something to consider. Medical school involves a transition from the relatively relaxed and responsibility light years of school and University life to the serious responsibilities of medical practice. Hanging on to the fun of learning, the excitement of clinical practice and the warm friendship of peers and team members must be encouraged and your education and associated assessments must not break any of this down. If it does your medical school and tutors will have failed you. However, medicine is a very serious business and the public expects the highest standards of professionalism from both clinically situated medical students and qualified doctors. Always arrive on time, dress smartly, leave any arrogance in the street, behave with a maturity beyond your years and be respectful of your tutors, the practice teams and especially the patients you meet. The assessment of professionalism is an increasingly important and explicit part of medical assessment – and primary care placements are particularly important settings in which to identify good and bad practice.

Formative assessment

Formative assessment is that part which doesn't contribute directly to the school allowing your progression into later years, or towards graduation. It is not less important for that. Formative is just that, aimed at 'forming' you, it is the 'educational core' of assessment. The formative assessments will be designed to help you benchmark, and reflect on, your progress and help you target your work effectively. It may give great insight into your interaction with patients or other staff, and into your development as a professional. If summatives are the hurdles you have to jump over, formative assessments are there to ensure you are fit and will be successful.

Your course handbook will outline your clinical science learning outcomes, the clinical skills you need to learn, and also talk about learning outcomes to do with the attitudes, values, and behaviours expected of the medical profession, that is, professionalism. The latter are difficult to teach, most are innate, but they are perhaps easier to assess (at least informally). Your primary care placements will often be longer than other placements on the course, or frequently offer continuity of relationship that doesn't always happen in other settings.

This gives an opportunity, especially on longitudinal placements, to enable a closer working with your tutor and in turn more authentic assessment not just of skills and competencies, but of the professional attributes essential in medicine. For this reason many students can find assessment and feedback on primary care/community placements particularly helpful and insightful. There is a counterargument which challenges the reliability, the validity and appropriateness of this process of assessment. Personality clashes, student or tutor problems, illness, a single unfortunate episode, diversity or cultural insensitivity etc., can create assessment bias. If you think that this may be developing or have happened, deal with it quickly with your tutor, your educational supervisor or the medical school faculty mechanisms at an early stage.

Formative assessment will range from the informal (direct comments on your performance against set benchmarks as you interact with staff and patients) to the formal. The formal may include all the range of assessments included in the section *How can you best use your time on primary care placements to survive (or even excel) in your medical school assessments?* The key thing is these are formative – take them seriously and take the chance to make them a positive experience.

Summative assessment

Summative assessments are those that directly affect progression or graduation. On your primary care placements these will include a mixture of reflection on professional practice perhaps backed up with portfolio, reflective diaries or reflective case discussions. You may have more formal workplace-based assessments. These may include direct observation of performance, often standardised and repeated (e.g., mini CEXs). Increasingly these will mirror the equivalent assessments you will encounter in early years as a junior doctor or primary care registrar. Much summative assessment will often be less based outside the placement and more focussed on the end of clinical block or end of year summative testing. This will use recognised standardised methods such as written examinations including multiple choice, single best answer or extending matching questions or, to asses clinical competencies, will use objective structured clinical examinations (OSCEs) or variants of long case examinations (e.g., OSLERs). In all these cases the assessment should be relevant to both your primary care- and secondary care-based learning experiences – and will, we hope, include common important cases you will frequently encounter within your primary care placements. They key point here is that assessment should reward the best students – and if you spend a lot of time with patients in primary care, exploring their problems and helping manage them, the assessment should be enjoyable and straightforward. Some schools have gone one step further and dropped specific high stakes end of year assessments to move to a wholly workplace-based assessment approach, in many ways this will further reward students who immerse themselves fully in workplace-based learning. 'Practice makes perfect' – or well thought out, guided practice with excellent tuition and feedback makes perfect. Make the most of the opportunities that come your way.

How can you best use your time on primary care placements to survive (or even excel) in your medical school assessments?

In the section, we've given some examples of where we believe your primary care placements can best prepare you for your medical school assessments. These examples are intended to show what can be very thoroughly covered in primary care, and those areas where we believe that primary care placements are uniquely positioned to drive your learning. The assessments mentioned may be used in both formative and summative ways.

Direct feedback on performance

Primary care placements have traditionally encouraged in-depth analysis of clinical and communication performance in the consultation, often using directly recorded patient encounters (e.g., use of 'videos' in postgraduate UK general practice training). If your teaching practice/placement has the equipment, embrace this opportunity – ask to be recorded. It can be of great educational value, especially with a supportive tutor to guide you through it. (NB: *Always make sure guidance on patient consent and information governance is being followed – with digital tapes erased after use*).

See also Chapter 4 on observed consultations for tips on how to maximise feedback on routine patient encounters.

Objective Structured Clinical Examinations (OSCE)

OSCEs are highly structured stations using clinical scenarios based on frequently encountered (and easily reproducible) patient problems. For that reasons primary care placements are a rich source of rehearsal. Ask your tutor to (a) practice introducing yourself to patients (b) taking focussed short histories – for example, respiratory, cardiac, abdominal (c) conducting focussed high-quality examinations – getting the basic right (the medical school will have guidance about what approach it likes – you and your tutor should be aware of this guidance) (d) giving advice – on self-care, on investigations, on treatment options (e) negotiating with patients about choices and decisions (f) summarising, handing over and explaining. You will get excellent teaching on all these elements if you ask – and especially in schools where your tutor helps with setting and conducting examinations. There is no better place than primary care to learn these skills and practice them – you just need to engage with your tutor and work with him/her and your colleagues.

Long cases, linked OSCE stations and Objective Structured Long Examination Record (OSLER)

Many schools have tried to link OSCEs together to offer students a more authentic long clinical scenario for assessment – with history-taking, examination and decision making combined. Others have retained 'long cases' or conduct OSLERs – which themselves are integrated longer patient cases.

Primary care placements are again a good place to gain the skills needed to make these examinations familiar and easy to excel at. Work with your tutor to practice, make sure you conduct at least one full consultation per week – observed and as you would in an examination (some time pressure, some hard questioning, honest objective informed feedback). At schools where your tutor examines (hopefully all cases) this will be second nature and welcomed – if it isn't, then discuss with your tutor about what is required. A particularly important ability is being able to cope with a patient who presents with more than one problem. That would be everyone of course. No patients have just one problem. Avoiding the panicky feeling in the examination when the patient starts to ramble and you start to flounder can only happen if you practice, practice, practice with the most physically, psychologically and socially complex people, such as those you will enjoy meeting in general practice.

Workplace-based assessments (WPBA)

These include a variety of tools – increasingly important in postgraduate clinical professional assessment. They include Mini-CEX, (Mini-Clinical Evaluation eXercise, a short oral examination based on a previously observed patient), DOPS (Direct Observation of Procedural Skills), CbD (Case-based Discussion), Mini-PAT (Mini-Peer Assessment Tool). All of these may be used in your primary care placement. They should be welcomed – they offer authentic assessment on real patients in real patient encounters.

Van der Vleuten and colleagues (2005) argued that when assessing professionals, the assessment methodologies should be designed fully integrated into the whole educational programme. They emphasise that repeated subjective evaluations can be appropriate and reliable. One of the great strengths of primary care placements is that you usually will have more direct sustained tutor contact, enabling this authentic assessment and informed feedback. At best your medical school will offer assessments which utilise longitudinal, workplace based embedded assessment processes (not just end of placement or end of year examinations). These judgement-based assessments are based on direct observation or reflection on clinical experiences, which are a valid, reproducible and increasingly an important assessment tool – and something you will encounter across postgraduate professional education. The challenge for a medical school is to ensure that their students achieve a safe and effective level of 'preparedness for practice', or 'Fitness to Practice'. It is important to understand this, how it increasingly shapes the assessments you will encounter, and understand why this makes your assessment within primary care a particularly rich source of information both for your own self-assessment of progress and for the medical school.

Using clinical portfolios in assessment

At best the assessments above will be combined into a reflective clinical portfolio – combining multiple sources of assessment and feedback with tutor feedback, patient feedback and your own self-reflection.

Such portfolios are complex, but at best offer rich sources of information for you and those educators seeking to support your journey into independent professional practice. Primary care placements, especially when longitudinal or integrated with secondary care, are an excellent place to have meaningful portfolios – for reasons previously discussed. Embrace their use if you get the chance.

Some potential strengths of assessment in primary care

In this section we will look at four areas where we believe primary care placements, especially longitudinal ones, have a real value in enhancing your education and in offering opportunity for an authentic assessment of progress and ability. Embrace these opportunities – and if you don't recognise them in your own school, use your student body or council to debate them with the school.

Longitudinal integrated clerkships and authentic assessments

Primary care placements offer the opportunity for creative approaches to the setting of learning objectives and teaching approaches for the assessments aligned to them. The development of longitudinal integrated clerkships offers the time for students to develop long-term associations with patients (Thistletwaite *et al.*, 2013). An example of this is the King's College London Community Study projects following a women through her pregnancy and her infant's first 3 months of life (Stephenson, 2012). Looking at health promotion activities or care improvement projects offers not only good education, but also allows excellent opportunities for meaningful assessment and feedback on performance in the workplace. These long-term relationship with patients are not confined to maternity – they have been used equally well in patients with new diagnoses of cancer, chronic diseases or mental health problems. The key point here is that all of them offer the chance to assess students learning about holistic care of patients (links between social, physical and mental health) and assessment about the skills to understand and care for patients with complex conditions and across multiple morbidities.

Learning and assessment from written work and projects

One area of learning and feedback we believe is often under-utilised in primary care is that of project work, audit and written work. The ability to write well is an essential skill, the ability to conduct small quality improvement reviews and projects or look in depth at a particular aspect of care is also essential for doctors. Many practices and primary care organisations will welcome support for looking at aspects of their clinical care – and will offer excellent supervision for such work. Seek out opportunities to align your expected work with your primary care placements – and make the most of the quality feedback that will be available.

Opportunities for such project work may arise within student selected components (SSCs), electives or research and audit or clinical improvement projects. Such SSCs and project work offer chances to assess and reinforce some vital skills for future practice in depth– skills such as teamworking, data gathering, writing skills, research skills, communication skills. Primary care has no monopoly on such skills – but does have an abundance of skilled tutors willing and able to teach and assess them.

Embedding learning about long-term conditions and multi-morbidity

Medicine is increasingly complicated with patients living longer, with more long-term conditions and ever more complicated multiple therapeutic interventions. It is rare for a 60-year-old patient to have no regular medication, and a majority of patients at 70 years have two of more long-term conditions and consume a plethora of drugs. We explored earlier how primary care is a good place to learn this complexity. It also follows that it is a sensible place to assess the knowledge, skills and approaches which help successful management of such patients – skills which include a patient-centred holistic approach, excellent communication, information gathering, risk assessment and excellent teamworking with a wide and expanding multi-professional healthcare team. The best medical schools already assess students in the workplace against the acquisition of such skills, and in doing so rightly reinforce their importance in your eyes. We believe all will follow suit soon, and the transition of assessment between undergraduate and postgraduate medicine will become more seamless than it currently is.

Assessing professionalism, principles and portfolios

The practice of medicine involves the acquisition of significant core knowledge, clinical competence and higher level thinking skills. The learning from the medical course must empower the students to become doctors able to apply skills and knowledge, analyse information, evaluate and measure its relevance, and then to formulate an appropriate diagnosis and management plan of care. In early clinical placements in primary care you will benefit from direct observation of the building blocks – the clinical skills, clinical history-taking and procedural skills needed to be competent and progress in your course. Tutors will also be working to encourage the learning and reinforce good professional principles – and these should form part of your assessment from the outset. In later years the learning which will be most readily tested in primary care will be to ensure that not only do you have the requisite knowledge and skills, but that you also possess the fundamental attitudes and values which will make you a safe and successful doctor. Are you ready for an increasingly independent professional practice? You should welcome these assessments, they should reassure you that you are where you want to be at your stage of the course, and your stage of the trajectory to becoming a doctor. Equally you should embrace opportunities for portfolio-based assessment – it will help reinforce skills you need to acquire for lifelong learning in an ever changing profession.

> **TIP**
>
> Assessment drives learning. As medical students you tend to learn what you are tested on, not the knowledge and skills you necessarily need as practicing clinicians. In the best medical schools the two will be closely aligned. If you think it is odd that your own school uses portfolios to assess your relationships with other professionals, or your approach to self-study, or other aspects of professionalism, remember this is because these will be crucial, may be 10–20 years later, when our understanding of physiology has changed or current drug treatments for disease are confined to museums.

TASK: A 15-MINUTE REFLECTION

We have talked a lot. Make a cup of tea, and put on your thinking caps. Chat with your fellow students.

Consider:

- How have my assessments so far helped or hindered my development?
- How I can best engage with assessments on this primary care placement to really learn about myself, my strengths and weaknesses?
- How can I ensure I end the placement as a better potential doctor than I started it?

TASK: SELF-REFLECTION AND SELF-AWARENESS

[With grateful acknowledgement to a variety of our own previous tutors].

At times in primary care you'll have time to think, may be during commuting to placement, within free time at lunch, or because the new perspectives it offers make you more receptive to do so. Many of us, the authors included, had real moments of insight and self-reflection on our medical student placements which influenced our subsequent career paths and indeed our lives.

Consider these questions:

1 Where am I?
2 Why am I in this position? (If you want to be somewhere else, you will have to do something differently: if you always do what you have always done, you will always get what you have always got.)
3 Where do I want to be?
4 Why do I want to be there?
5 What do I have to do?
6 What blocks do I have to overcome?

The first point is self-assessment, the second self-awareness, the third is wisdom (but also laid out in your course handbooks), the fourth is your motivation, the fifth and sixth will be influenced by your learning ability and maturity. These are the six *strategic* questions of life and can apply equally to plan your next placement, your next five years, repairing a bicycle or developing government health strategy. Use your primary care placement to reflect on these questions, ideally with your colleagues on placement. You could also reflect with your tutor – who may find it personally useful (there are many advantages to having medical students in the practice!).

Opportunities for self-assessment in primary care settings

Possessing self-awareness through a robust and regular self-assessment of where you need to be (in the domains of knowledge, skills and professional attitudes), alongside a level of integrity that allows you to happily have discussions about weaknesses and failures is exactly what society wants in their medical students and their doctors. You must never stop learning to be a good doctor, and you cannot continue learning without reflection and self-assessment. Use your primary care placements to hone these skills – you will be well guided and such assessment is what drives continued professional development for your clinical tutors.

The concept of good self-assessment is aligned with the principles of any good quality assessment and involves 'validity; that is, judging your performance against appropriate criteria (e.g., performing high quality self-examinations) and 'accuracy', that is gaining reasonable concurrence between self-claimed and other validated measures of performance (Gordon, 1991). You can see this as contributing to your professionalisation, embedding and aligning your behaviours with those of your future peers. Self-assessment, though based on a paradigm of reflective practice is more than this. You should identify standards, and criteria, however implicitly, and then make judgements, or formally test the extent to which you have met these standards. Ideally all committed to a learning portfolio. Hence the exercise smoothly links to the postgraduate world of career progression, lifelong learning, appraisal and revalidation.

There is evidence which shows consistently that your student peers, and the school's faculty, will often make more valid and favourable assessments of your performance than you do of yourself (BEME *et al.*, 2008). Make sure any self-assessment is well informed and accurate; it is best done with the guidance of your tutor, especially within the longitudinal placements encountered in primary care.

Some final thoughts: why authenticity in assessment matters

Although you and your tutors have objectives, and assessment of your ability to achieve competence could reasonably be a purely objective exercise, as we have discussed your tutors will also apply their professional judgement in assessing you. This is subjective, open to challenge of credibility and validity. How you perform in displaying your knowledge, skills and behaviours, attitudes and values in the programmed 'tests' is important to your tutors in forming a judgement about you, but we argue that they will often be less valuable to you than the end of placement grades and associated feedback. The GP tutor has a significant responsibility to help you achieve your required learning outcomes, but what will really keep him or her awake at night is the risk they are managing on behalf of society in allowing you to progress to become a doctor, a member of their own profession, if you are not fit. They will therefore assess you rigorously.

Feedback within your primary care placement

> Good feedback will be effective in improving learning and performance
>
> GMC TD (2009b) Supplementary Guidance
> on Assessment Para 126

This statement, as we discussed in the section on formative assessment, is probably an understatement of what you will already be aware is at the heart of good teaching. The best teachers have a great skill – of being able to reflect back on your performance, benchmark it against where you have come from and where you should be and let you know how to improve without deflating you. We can all learn, we can all improve –as clinicians we all have to keep learning and improving. It is part of our professional duties, and of course essential in a fast-changing environment. The power of feedback in education is based on its centrality and frequency. The tutor can only give feedback from a position of credibility and respect. The tutor should embark on an appropriate student-centred respectful dialogue, eliciting your thoughts and feelings, stressing the elements of good performance and delivering difficult messages constructively and thoughtfully. The best tutors will also be a facilitator of learning – encouraging feedback from your peers, other staff members and patients.

The issue of feedback by tutors to medical students, as adult learners, is often a cause of concern for the school and students alike. Students usually feel (a) it is not done enough and (b) the quality isn't high enough. In general, primary care placements buck this trend and have a reputation for excellent feedback, often more valid as tutors are more visible and with you for longer.

> **TASK**
>
> Talk with your primary care tutor at an early stage and make it clear you'd like feedback on your performance, and not just as part of the formative and summative assessments.
>
> Ask your tutor to highlight how you are doing on your journey to becoming a doctor.
>
> Ask them to be honest in highlighting where you have bypassed an important area of learning and may risk failure in summative assessments.

This is a book about community and primary care placements. What is different about feedback in this environment? In many ways, nothing, – but we believe it just happens more frequently and tends to be more personal and relevant. The principles of good feedback are constant across different clinical settings, and we have tried to provide our own summary of these in Box 9.1.

The authors experience, and that stated by their students, is that feedback is often at its most effective within primary care placements. A variety of explanations may account for this:

1   Feedback should ideally be based on direct observation or interaction with a student. This does not always happen, but because of the

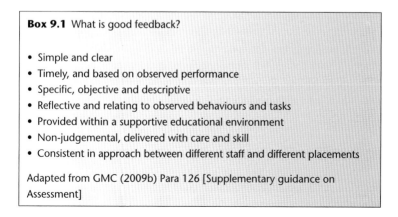

> **Box 9.1** What is good feedback?
>
> • Simple and clear
> • Timely, and based on observed performance
> • Specific, objective and descriptive
> • Reflective and relating to observed behaviours and tasks
> • Provided within a supportive educational environment
> • Non-judgemental, delivered with care and skill
> • Consistent in approach between different staff and different placements
>
> Adapted from GMC (2009b) Para 126 [Supplementary guidance on Assessment]

nature of community placements (often with individual tuition) it is much more likely. Ask your tutor for feedback if it's not volunteered.

2 Many placements in primary care offer longitudinal personalised contact with a named tutor, allowing for the chance for informed, comprehensive and constructive feedback. You should recognise and seek that opportunity.

3 Many placements in primary care offer the chance to reflect on a very wide range of interactions with a variety of patients and colleagues (a greater variety than for example on a more specialised hospital ward, especially as hospital stays becomes shorter and pressure on beds ever greater). This allows informed tutor feedback on a range of skills, plus the chance of multisource feedback from different health professionals and a range of patients.

4 Genuine feedback from patients, their carers or families may be more readily available in community settings. Patients are voluntary, often more empowered than in hospital and usually less acutely ill.

Types of feedback in primary care placements

Feedback from your tutor

Much of your feedback in primary care will be directly via your tutor, often but not always a GP. GPs possess a wealth of operational medical knowledge and skills, and of course ingrained professional abilities and values, but are usually lacking in the full range of detailed specialist clinical and technical knowledge. Feedback will therefore *tend* to be tailored in respect of the former, less so against the latter, but understanding the limits of GP knowledge is helpful learning in its own right. The tutor's ability to freely admit their ignorance of certain issues (and share how they manage this) is itself a feedback about themselves to you which is an interesting twist. You should value and seek feedback even if you know you have done well. Aim to be as good a clinician as you possibly can. Always ask for *specific advice* on what you can do to be a little bit better, even when you get praised in general terms. A pat on the back is always nice, a focussed clear helpful piece of guidance will stay with you longer.

Feedback from peers

Another great source of feedback on your primary care placements will be your peers. During your time at medical school you will learn informally and formally with your peers – but be aware this learning never stops, certainly not at graduation. On your primary care placements you will often be in groups, perhaps travelling together long distances, often paired together for a long time. This can be tricky – but equally make the most of the educational opportunity it brings. Work in pairs or groups. Observe each other seeing patients, or presenting patient stories. Learn from colleagues, seek their feedback 'Be honest – what did I do well, what could I have done better?' – give feedback, you will learn from that too (*see also section giving and receiving feedback*).

Feedback from more senior colleagues and 'near peers'

Another potential strength in your primary care placement is obtaining feedback from more senior students attached to the practice ('near peers'), colleagues who have just graduated (e.g., Foundation Year 2 doctors in UK settings – most of whom do primary care rotations) and from those on general practice/family medicine speciality training programmes (Dick *et al.*, 2007; Kirby *et al.*, 2014; Rushforth *et al.*, 2010). In primary care longer placements often mean you'll get to know these colleagues better than you would in hospital placements. This in turn allows more chance for meaningful feedback from those only a little way ahead of you on your journey to be a doctor.

Multisource (or 360 degree) feedback

Many medical schools are actively encouraging multisource feedback or '360 degree' feedback. In the United Kingdom *Tomorrow's Doctors* requires medical schools to learn with and about other professionals; GMC (2009a) TD *Para 22 a–d*. Assessment drives learning. It is inevitable that where students know their colleagues from other professions will be assessing them as well as teaching them they will take those aspects of their studies more seriously. We hope that applies to you – learn to understand and respect the roles of your professional colleagues (practice nurses, nurse practitioners, health visitors, community pharmacist etc.) and consider yourself fortunate if they are encouraged to take the time to give you feedback – it will be valuable in your growth and development as a doctor.

Feedback from patients

> Ensure that you seek feedback about your performance from patients
> or carers after contact with a patient in a learning setting
>
> Tomorrows Doctors 2009; Para 111 (GMC, 2009a)

The UK's General Medical Council has urged medical schools to use patients actively in student learning, including a role in assessment and feedback (GMC, 2009b, c). Many schools do. Some have interpreted this as involving specific high level interventions, often with 'expert patients' – the highest grade of Towle's hierarchy of patient involvement (Towle *et al.*, 2010). We believe one important role of community and primary care based medical education is to give a voice in education to the 'ordinary' patient.

We have two reasons:

1 Patients in primary care are empowered – they book their appointment, they are often fairly well, they are in their own clothes, they feel in control. As such they are ideally placed to tell their stories, and in turn give their informed opinions.

2 Patients in these settings very often (ideally always) consent specifically to seeing the medical students, often at the time of booking their appointment. Perhaps as a result (in our experience) they always seem more than willing to help and go the extra mile – including giving personal feedback on student progress.

Both these things mean patient feedback in this setting is particularly valuable.

TASK

At best your tutors should prompt the patient after each encounter:
'OK – just before you go, are you able to tell James/Jasmine one thing they did well, and one thing they could have done to make them a better doctor'.
Powerful, immediate, impartial feedback. Ask your tutor to try it.
If it isn't happening, do it yourself, for example, if you are with the patient and waiting for the tutor to reappear, try asking: 'How did I do? What could I do better? Was my explanation clear? Is there anything I should have asked? What makes a good doctor?'
You will be amazed at the comments – and their effects on your performance.
Never miss a chance to learn from and with patients.

Feedback from carers and family members

The other group you will have access to on your primary care placements is the families, partners or carers of patients you see. Obviously this is true often in hospital – but again in primary care you have the benefit of empowerment (patients book appointments, they are not admitted or referred as in hospital), wellness (often patients are continuing with normal lives, albeit carrying chronic illnesses), context (patients are brought in my concerned carers or relatives or friends) and time (not always, but often a useful factor on home visits, with mothers and children or more elderly patients).

Involve the carers and relatives – learn from them, but also seek feedback from them:

> 'What would you like your Dad's doctor to do to best help him?' or 'What advice would you have for me as I seek to become a better doctor?'

Giving and receiving feedback

Finally, don't forget it is also extremely good practice as well as personally beneficial to become skilled at giving feedback. This in turn will help you reflect on your own emotions when you receive it. When you give feedback to colleagues follow the rules given in Box 9.1 (What is good feedback?). Ensure it is constructive, based on specific examples of behaviour and suggests options to improve. 'Colin, in my opinion you gave a really good general summary to the patient, but I wonder if she might have felt criticised when you mentioned weight loss; could you have phrased it different – for example by saying xxxxxx'. Practice doing this. You will learn, your colleagues will learn, they will reciprocate – and you will gain skills of summarising as well as being forced to be more attentive when others are doing the work!

As you do this you'll come back to learning more about yourself. Receiving feedback itself is an art – listen to the specifics, concentrate on your behaviour and its effect on others – and if it is too general or unhelpful challenge it – after all it is your degree and your career (and in many countries your financial commitment)!

Giving something back – your responsibility to offer feedback

The previous sections of this chapter have been about you. How can you best use assessment to become a better doctor? How can you encourage constructive feedback and use it to your advantage? This final section is about your professional responsibility to get involved with making medical education better and making clinical practice better. Students, and all health professionals, must contribute to quality assurance processes in education and in clinical practice. In the United Kingdom the failures were recently uncovered across a number of care indicators at Mid-Staffordshire Foundation Trust hospitals, and the subsequent inquiry (Francis Report, 2013) highlighted the roles students and those in professional training should play in future in highlighting concerns relating to patient safety, and led to the introduction of a statutory 'Duty of Candour' of relevance to you both now and after graduation (DoH, 2014).

TASK

Discuss with your colleagues and your tutor:
How can you help make your placement better for those who come next?
How can you help your placement provider to improve clinical care?
What role might you play in helping highlight concerns about clinical care – and how could this be done carefully and sensitively?

Educational standards and quality assurance

As a medical student you have a very important formal role to play in evaluating and improving the quality of the placements you experience. This will help future students, help your tutors develop as educators, help the practice develop as a teaching practice (for students and other learners.) Practices will value and seek out this feedback – tutors use it for their NHS appraisal, practices for their quality assurance (increasingly a formal requirement of accreditation and contracts). Medical schools will have formal student feedback processes in operation and use the data, for example, to prepare for their statutory quality assurance visits.

Quality assurance of placements

Good tutors will ask how you found the educational experience, how you found their teaching. Good Schools will ensure you are empowered to give you tutors individualised constructive feedback – and ensure the best teacher gets the praise, plaudits and awards they deserve. Don't underestimate your power to motivate and enthuse your teachers and help reward those that go the extra mile. Much of education is hard work, and time for teaching and supervision is badly squeezed by clinical pressures – make time to ensure it is rewarded by positive feedback. Such feedback also feeds into the overall School quality assurance processes, its returns to the General Medical Council (United Kingdom) or equivalent bodies and will be used within external quality assurance visits (e.g., QAA in UK Universities).

Where a placement did not go as well, your role is even more important, albeit trickier. Your medical school should encourage and support you in giving honest feedback without fear of it affecting grades. You have a professional duty to give this feedback. Consider what we said above: comment on behaviour or actions you found unhelpful, give specific examples, give positive suggestions for improvement. Think of the most useful feedback you have received and seek to replicate it (in terms of approach). This feedback should go direct to the practice and tutor, and if anything other than minor concerns should go also to the medical school placement organiser (follow your own School's advice). If you are really stuck and don't know what to do if a placement gave cause for concern, ask you student representatives for advice, or talk to your personal tutor.

Remember in all this there is no place for anonymous or scurrilous feedback – you are now a professional and have a duty to give constructive measured objective advice and offer examples of concern – the same standards you'd expect of any concerns raised about your own standards or behaviour.

Quality assurance of teaching practices

Cotton *et al.* (2009) explored with a range of professionals and students the requirements of a teaching practice – these have helped all medical schools set clear standards which should be available to you as students and form the basis of your feedback and assessment of your learning experience. Medical schools use your feedback to improve the quality of teaching and ensure the set learning objectives are being met. In UK schools this is now a formal part of accreditation with the GMC (End of Placement Survey), albeit as authors we have concerns that this survey data is often not specific to the primary care placements which sometimes appear as an afterthought. Giving both verbal and written feedback are skills that you need to learn. Medical schools should ensure that you understand the outcomes of any feedback that you have given such as curricular changes, and schools use a variety of methods to do this such as information pages on virtual learning sites, staff–student liaison committees and conferences. Closing the feedback loop is an important stage and of course encourages you to give feedback in the first place. Encourage the School to do this – and talk to student representatives if you feel more could be done.

Focus groups in some UK medical schools, reflecting on students' involvement in quality assurance showed that they believed patients should have a more direct role in student education and quality assurance (Macallan and Pearson, 2013). You might have similar insights and ideas to share with the placement provider, practice or School. If you are really keen, or the School takes this very seriously, other tools are available to assess the educational environment, for example, the Dundee Readiness for Educational Environment Measure (DREEM). Talk to the practice or tutor about using this as an alternative framework with which to give student feedback on the placement, or consider it as an audit project if you have one to do.

Clinical care and clinical governance, what role can you play?

One motivation for clinicians volunteering to teach is to maintain their enthusiasm and 'keep them on their toes'. You are part of that. Asking questions helps maintain the enthusiasm of your tutors, and in turn helps raise standards of clinical care. What is the most useful role you can play in helping drive up clinical standards? This is likely to take one of three forms.

- First you have a duty as a whistleblower to give specific feedback (NOT anonymous) if you are concerned about serious unprofessional practice (Francis Report, 2013). This is a responsibility, and one to take very seriously and remember to seek advice if at all unsure of what you might have witnessed – what may appear to you to be flippant or unprofessional may be completely acceptable in the context of a long-term doctor–patient relationship.

• Second, you may have non-specific concerns about the conduct, health or well-being of a clinician you work with – you should act on these concerns and ensure you mention these concerns to your tutor or the practice manager (as a professional colleague, not a spy).

• Third, you may have positive suggestions and ideas for change, something you have seen work well elsewhere, or new clinical and therapeutic advances from your study or time in hospital. Share these.

As we stated earlier – never underestimate the positive role you can play in healthcare provision even from your early days in medical school. Having enthusiastic, interested and engaged medical students help motivate your tutors and is much liked by patients who feel they get better listened to, and aside from that like to 'give something back'. Use this positive influence wisely.

Summary

So – you survived a chapter on assessment, feedback and quality assurance – or maybe you were just strategic and read the introductions and summary! We hope you have learned a little of assessment in general, a little of its application in primary care placements and how it can drive the learning of complex professional practice as well as simpler easily measured objectives. We hope you have come to look forward to decent authoritative informed personal feedback, something that should be a real strength of these placements. We hope you have considered your own opportunities to give feedback, and help influence the development of high quality educational and clinical practice. Finally we hope you better understand your role and responsibilities in quality assurance and the enhancement of education in primary care and indeed clinical work in primary care. Perhaps you may even have become a little inspired to get more involved in this vital area.

References

BEME; Colthart, I.; Bagnall, G.; Evans, A.; Allbutt, H.; Haig, A.; Illing, J.; McKinstry, B. (2008) The effectiveness of self-assessment on the identification of learner needs, learner activity, and impact on clinical practice: BEME guide 10. Medical Teacher 30(2): 124–145.

Cotton, P.; Sharp, D.; Howe, A.; Starkey, C.; Laue, B.; Hibble, A.; Benson, J. (2009) Developing a set of quality criteria for community-based medical education in the UK. Education for Primary Care 20: 143–151.

Dick, M.L.B.; King, D.B.; Mitchell, G.K.; Kelly, G.D., Buckley, J.F.; Garside, S.J. (2007) Vertical integration in learning and teaching (VITAL): an approach to medical education in general practice. Medical Journal of Australia 187(2): 133–135.

DoH (2014) Requirements for registration with the Care Quality Commission: response to consultations on fundamental standards, the Duty of Candour and the fit and proper persons requirement for directors Department of Health, London. http://www.gmc-uk.org/static/documents/content/DoC_guidance_englsih.pdf. Accessed 7 July 2015.

Francis Report (2013) Final Report of the Mid Staffordshire NHS Trust Public Inquiry. http://www.midstaffspublicinquiry.com/report. Accessed 18 March 2015.

Gordon, M.J. (1991) A review of the validity and accuracy of self-assessments in health professions training. Academic Medicine 66: 762–769.

GMC (2009a) Tomorrow's Doctors. http://www.gmc-uk.org/static/documents/content/Tomorrows_Doctors_1214.pdf. Accessed 23 March 2015.

GMC (2009b) Tomorrow's doctors supplementary advice – assessment in undergraduate medical education. http://www.gmc-uk.org/Assessment_in_undergraduate_medical_education_1114.pdf_56439668.pdf. Accessed 23 March 2015.

GMC (2009c) Patient and public involvement in undergraduate medical education advice supplementary to Tomorrow's Doctors 2009. Available at: http://www.gmc-uk.org/static/documents/content/Patient_and_public_involvement_in_undergraduate_medical_education_1114.pdf. Accessed 7 July 2015.

Kirby, J.; Rushforth, B.; Nagel, C.; Pearson, D.J. (2014) Should GP specialty trainees teach? Contrasting views from GP specialty trainees and their trainers. Education for Primary Care 25: 96–102.

Macallan, J.; Pearson, D. (2013) Medical student perspectives of what makes a high quality teaching practice. Education for Primary Care 24(3): 195–201.

Rushforth, B.; Kirby, J.; Pearson, D.J. (2010) General practice registrars as teachers: a review of the literature. Education for Primary Care 21: 221–229.

Stephenson, A. (2012) Kings Undergraduate Medical Education in the Community Report. Kings College, London. 2011–2012.

Thistlethwaite, J.; Bartle, E.; Chong, A.; Dick, M.; King, D.; Mahoney, S.; Papinczak, T.; Tucker, G. (2013) The effectiveness of longitudinal community placements in medical education BEME guide 26. Medical Teacher 2013: e1340–e1364

Towle, A.; Bainbridge, L.; Godolphin, W.; Katz, A.; Kline, C.; Lown, B.; Madularu, I.; Solomon, P.; Thistlethwaite, J. (2010) Active patient involvement in the education of health professionals. Medical Education 44: 64–74.

van der Vleuten, C.P.M.; Schuwirth, L.W.T (2005) Assessing professional competence: from methods to programmes. Medical Education 39: 309–317.

Chapter 10 **Conclusions: Looking to the future**

We hope very much you have enjoyed the book. We hope you are able to consult it throughout your time at medical school. We hope it will inform and enhance your primary care and community placements through stimulating discussion with your colleagues and your tutors.

Our own objectives in writing this book were simple. We wanted all students to have the best chance to experience the very high quality teaching that we have seen in primary care, and avoid the occasional lapses in standards, which still occurs. We also wanted to point out that much of what you need to learn to become a doctor needs to be learned within a community context because of the significant changes that are occurring in the NHS and across all health systems worldwide.

We'll finish with some personal thoughts from the two main authors. We are experienced tutors closely involved with educational and political developments in the field, and are both still active as general medical practitioners and tutors. That doesn't mean we have any more ability to see the future than you or our colleagues – but we have some insight and ideas about what you might expect in this field in the future.

Read our dialogue:

DAVID: So Sandra, what have we missed out and what will look outdated in 5 years' time if we are asked to revise this book?

SANDRA: The way we as healthcare professionals deliver care to our most needy patients, those with multiple co-morbidities

How to Succeed on Primary Care and Community Placements, First Edition.
David Pearson and Sandra Nicholson.
© 2016 John Wiley & Sons, Ltd. Published 2016 by John Wiley & Sons, Ltd.

living in areas of social deprivation, for example, will change. The current structures often presenting silos of social, health and educational support will be better integrated and our students will need to experience and learn from these opportunities. I genuinely believe that more and more health needs will be met within community settings in the United Kingdom and elsewhere and what we will see is ultimately undergraduate healthcare students spending the majority of their time within community settings. How technology and communication systems will facilitate this will need to be revised, I suspect.

DAVID: And, what do you think the next big things are? If it helps let me pitch in with an initial thought

I can see a return to a more hands-on educational approach. Students will increasingly be asked to participate and contribute to work during their primary care placements. The reason I loved my own primary care placements, in Edinburgh, very many years ago, was because I sat in the GP's chair – I did the consultations and I felt useful. I think this will increasingly be a model – especially perhaps in allowing medical schools to give something back to the communities and patients who support the education of their students. Students may be encouraged or expected to provide services for hard-to-reach communities, at antisocial hours or at times of stress in the service. Provided the supervision is excellent, the placements are truly educational and the patients are protected – why not?

SANDRA: The changes in doctors' working hours and the introduction of shifts within the UK NHS has significantly affected not only continuity of patient care, but also how students feel attached to 'firms'. Encouraging students to engage and truly participate in their own learning is one of today's major medical education challenges. Much of what you suggest depends (in the United Kingdom at least) on how the 'Greenaway report' (Shape of Training, 2013) is implemented which encourages us to think about how best to prepare medical students for full registration as doctors immediately following graduation. Many of the examples of good opportunities for learning while on community placements provide scope for greater student participation in service delivery, prioritising generalism and ensuring medical students are ready to work with all the required professional and practical skills.

OK, let me ask you something now: we've included chapters on technology and social media.

Why so?

DAVID: We have said a little about virtual learning and social media – but clearly these are areas which will assume greater significance in education, educational support and assessment in the next 5 years. I think we are only just taking off – and I can see community placements embracing the increasing use of technology in education. Why? Because it will have to, otherwise students and clinicians will get isolated and get left behind. Expect much greater integration of learning, online communities of educational practice, sophisticated online self-assessment and progress testing and electronic portfolios with multisource assessments as standard.

SANDRA: One of the community's major strengths is in its tutor expertise. Students have repeatedly benefitted from not only excellent clinical exposure and meeting a variety of patients while on placements, but also the consistent and often individual supervision received from their tutors. Good feedback requires direct observation of a student's performance. Many GP tutors are also inspirational role models. Would you not agree David?

DAVID: Absolutely – and I think they are inspirational because they fundamentally believe in the importance of what they are doing – as generalists in medicine looking after not only their patients in a holistic way, but also in their roles as educators (something going back to the days of Hippocrates).

Let me finish with a prediction. I think primary care will find its niche as two current educational ideas come together: team-based learning within longitudinal multi-professional clerkships. First, we need team-based learning – as future practice will be all about sophisticated team work to meet patients' increasingly complex needs. Second, the clear advantages of longitudinal placements will be aligned with the obvious potential of community placements – a reputation for skilled, well trained and committed tutors and the flexibility to offer long placements with continuity of supervision. The potential for remarkable learning will be there where these meet – the challenge for clinical academics like us will be to encourage, capture and disseminate such learning.

SANDRA: Yes, longitudinal integrated clerkships are certainly educationally inspiring and it's hard to see without general practice at their heart how these can operate successfully (at least in the United Kingdom). There are so many aspects of professional practice that community placements can help students learn about, but the centrality and therapeutic nature of the doctor–patient relationship and the value of effective teamwork for high quality patient care seems like a good place to start.

DAVID: …and if I can add one more, I would pitch for increased patient participation in learning. I hope we will see increased education, training and reward for those patients involved with primary care education, especially those with long-term conditions who we'll call on repeatedly for teaching and assessment, and who bring a true and profound insight into the effect of their health conditions on their lives (and the lives of their friends and families). Perhaps we should dedicate this book to them, and hope it makes a difference to their future care?

Reference

Shape of Training (2013). Securing the future of excellent patient care final report of the independent review Led by Professor David Greenaway. http://www.shapeoftraining.co.uk/static/documents/content/Shape_of_training_FINAL_Report.pdf_53977887.pdf (accessed 22 March 2015).

Index

Locators in **bold** refer to figures and tables

How to Succeed on Primary Care and Community Placements, First Edition.
David Pearson and Sandra Nicholson.
© 2016 John Wiley & Sons, Ltd. Published 2016 by John Wiley & Sons, Ltd.

pitfalls. *see* what can go wrong
placements
   author dialogues 194–7
   quality assurance 189
portfolios 12, 13, 52, 105, 176–7, 179
postnatal care 121–2
post-publication peer-review 153
poverty 9–11, 33. *see also* psycho-
   social determinants of health
practical skills enhancement. *see*
   procedural skills
practice manager roles **93**
practice nurses **91**, 98–9
practice-based healthcare teams. *see*
   primary healthcare teams
pregnancy **92**, 121–2
preparation for community
   placements xiii, 42–5, 60
   active learning 54–6
   on arrival 47–8
   health and safety 46, 50–1
   learning how to behave as a
     doctor 56–9
   personal learning plans and
     goals 53–4
   practical considerations 50–2
   professionalism 48–50
   reviewing the experience/review
     meetings 59–60
   travel planning 45–6, 51
preparedness for practice,
   assessment 176, 182
prescribing
   clinical information
     systems 139–41
   later years placements 23–5
   learning from pharmacists 100–4
   see also medicines
preventive medicine 36–9. *see also*
   public health

primary healthcare team
   placements xi, xiii, 85–7, 90
   clinical skills
     enhancement 95–8, **96–7**
   further resources 110
   learning from mistakes 106
   pharmacists 100–4
   practice nurses 98–9
   professionalism **87**, 87–8
   role in medical education 107–9
   roles 90, **91–4**
   shadowing professionals 95
   team meetings 105–6
   teamworking 88–90
proactive approaches. *see* active
   learning
problems. *see* what can go wrong
procedural skills 3
   direct observation 176
   early years placements 11–13
   medical school
     curriculum **96–7**
   in primary healthcare teams 85,
     86, 95–8, **96–7**
professional development xiii,
   144
professionalism
   assessment 171–2, 179
   digital 151, 155
   learning how to behave as a
     doctor 5–8, 56–9
   preparation for community
     placements 48–50
   primary healthcare teams **87**,
     87–8
   quality assurance 189
   teamworking attitudes 89
profiles, online 151, 155
projects. *see* research projects
psychiatric nurses, roles **92**